Helping Your Anxious Child

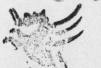
Dr David Lewis has specialised in treating anxiety and phobia conditions in adults and children for more than ten years. A lecturer in psychopathology at the University of Sussex, he is a founding trustee of Action on Phobias, a charity helping anxiety-sufferers of all ages, and a clinical director of Stresswatch, a non-profit-making organisation which advises industry on stress-related problems.

'Full of calm common sense about diagnosing anxieties and coping with them, especially those associated with school: taking exams, making friends and enemies, learning maths.'

Times Educational Supplement

Helping Your
Anxious Child

AN EFFECTIVE TREATMENT
FOR CHILDHOOD FEARS

David Lewis

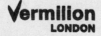

Vermilion
LONDON

9 10

Copyright © 1988 David Lewis

David Lewis has asserted his moral right to be identified as
the author of this work in accordance with the Copyright,
Design and Patents Act 1988.

First published in 1988 by Methuen, London
This edition published in the United Kingdom in 2002 by
Vermilion,
an imprint of Ebury Press
Random House UK Ltd.
Random House
20 Vauxhall Bridge Road
London SW1V 2SA

Addresses for companies within the Random House Group Limited can be
found at: www.randomhouse.co.uk/offices.htm

Random House UK Limited Reg. No. 954009
www.randomhouse.co.uk
A CIP catalogue record is available for this book from the
British Library.

ISBN 9780091884338

Penguin Random House is committed to a sustainable future for
our business, our readers and our planet. This book is made from
Forest Stewardship Council® certified paper.

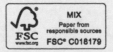

MIX
Paper from
responsible sources
FSC® C018179

Printed and bound in Great Britain by Clays Ltd, St Ives plc

To my mother
with love and gratitude

Contents

Acknowledgements   ix
Introduction   xi

Part One: Why your child gets anxious
1 Your anxious child   3
2 Your questions answered   17
3 Why your child gets anxious   26
4 Your child's hidden fears   42

Part Two: Exploring your child's anxieties
5 Discovering your child's anxieties   61
6 Exploring your child's anxieties   74
7 Pinpointing specific anxieties   93
8 Discovering your own anxieties   99

Part Three: Banishing your child's anxieties
9 How to help your anxious child   109
10 The relaxation response   115

Part Four: Helping with specific anxieties
11 Helping your child with social anxiety   139
12 Helping to banish maths anxiety   156
13 Helping achieve exam success   171
14 Helping your phobic child   187
15 Helping your social anxiety   201
16 Helping with sexual anxiety   206

Part Five: Living without anxiety
17 Living without anxiety   219

   Bibliography   225
   Index   237

Acknowledgements

I should like to express my grateful thanks to the many hundreds of parents and children who have been working with the procedures described in this book, and providing such invaluable feedback and encouragement. My thanks too to my research associate Shandy Mathias, BSc, for her continued support and involvement in these studies. Finally, my thanks to artist Richard Armstrong, who created Dibs as well as producing the other illustrations in this book.

Introduction

This is the part of the book most people usually skip, but I ask you to take a few moments to read it, because it is going to help you make the most of what follows.

Since this is a practical book, intended to help you solve a practical problem – your child's anxieties, phobias or fears – it should not be read as one would a novel or detective story. There is no need to start at the first page and read in sequence to the last one. You can, of course, do this if you wish. But if your main purpose is to extract the facts needed to assist your child as quickly as possible, here's how I suggest you approach the content.

The book is divided into five parts. Chapters One to Four explain the nature of anxiety, what it is, how it arises and the various guises it may assume in your child's life. These chapters will help you understand the how and why of anxious feelings, so making it easier to appreciate the way in which fears can strike, their effect on performance, and why the practical procedures I describe can prove so effective. Although the subject is a technical one, I am confident that you will find the material easy to follow.

Like the rest of the book, the content of these chapters is based not only on clinical experience and research, but also on the talks which I have presented to thousands of parents in Europe and the USA over many years. Unlike the unfortunate reader, who if anything proves incomprehensible has no one to turn to for guidance, lecture audiences can and do protest if explanations are confused or confusing. I hope, therefore, that needless complexity and unnecessary jargon has been thoroughly purged from the text. If you do get stuck, then write to me and I'll try and help. Unlike many authors who regard corresponding with readers as a chore to be avoided, I welcome your views, suggestions, comments and queries. Please e-mail me at mail@lewisandleyser.com

Chapters Five to Eight are concerned with ways of discovering whether your child's difficulties really are due to anxiety and, if so, which areas of his or her life are responsible.

To conduct these investigations I have developed a number of questionnaires. While such assessments can prove very helpful, they should never be taken as providing the final word on your child's feelings. No assessment, administered at a distance through the pages of a book, can do more than provide a general indication of what may be going wrong. You should regard them not as a thermometer giving a precise temperature reading, but as a litmus paper which, by changing colour, tells one whether a substance is acid or alkaline and offers a general indication of the strength, but nothing more.

Such tests have a number of inherent weaknesses, as any psychometrician – the name given to psychologists who specialise in creating tests – will confirm. One of these is an understandable tendency to 'fake good' when responding. That is, to provide not an honest answer but one which shows you in the best possible light, or supplies the kind of information it is believed that the person setting the test would wish to hear. For instance, if you were applying for a job in door-to-door selling and were asked, 'Would you sooner stay at home and listen to quiet music or attend a lively party?' it doesn't take an Einstein to guess that saying 'attend a lively party' will enhance your chances of landing the job.

One can get around this, to some extent, by using what are called 'projective tests'. Here the subject is presented with an ambiguous drawing or design – the most famous of these tests is probably the Rorschach Ink Blot – and asked to read a meaning into it.

Unfortunately, the range of possible answers is so wide that the responses can only be interpreted on a one-to-one basis by qualified testers – and even then many psychologists would argue that they are unreliable. In the course of my researches into childhood anxiety, I have developed a form of assessment that combines an element of projection – your child will be asked to put himself or herself in the place of a comic strip character – with a set of responses that can be more easily marked. It has proved a useful assessment that can give a good indication of both levels of anxiety and the areas of life in which these seem to be occurring. But, like all tests, it is not 100 per cent perfect, so use the information it provides as a sketch map of the emotional areas being explored, rather than as the definitive guide.

Chapters Nine and Ten contain practical procedures for bringing the mental and physical symptoms of anxiety under control. I regard these as the essential foundations on which this home-help plan for anxieties is constructed. This makes these two chapters, in many ways, the most crucial in the book. The sooner you start working on the procedures they contain the better.

Chapters Eleven to Sixteen explore different areas of anxiety which, in my professional experience, cause the greatest difficulties for children. Deciding which of these to read will depend on the type of problems your child is currently experiencing. The assessments will assist in identifying these areas. For example:

Anxiety caused by	*Read and use*
Attending School	Chapter Eleven
Doing Sums	Chapter Twelve
Taking Exams	Chapter Thirteen
A Phobia	Chapter Fourteen
Social Activities	Chapter Fifteen
Sex	Chapter Sixteen

Finally, in Chapter Seventeen, I explain how to go forward once you have helped your child banish his or her anxieties and fears. This chapter should, therefore, be read no matter what specific difficulty your child has been experiencing.

Part One
Why your child gets anxious

One
Your Anxious Child

My purpose in writing this book is to give you a simple and effective means of helping overcome your child's anxieties, phobias and fears. The procedures I am going to describe have been developed from clinical research and my personal experience in treating anxiety-sufferers of all ages.

You will find this book of great practical value if your child has:

- A general anxiety problem. This may reveal itself in a reluctance to attempt anything new, a strong dislike of change and an unwillingness to try his or her hand at unfamiliar tasks.
- A specific phobia, for instance of spiders, birds, dogs, or cats, sufficiently intense to prevent him or her from doing the kinds of things that children normally undertake without difficulty.
- Problems in class due to excessive anxiety. This may be making it hard for him to understand a specific subject, for instance arithmetic, or for her to achieve her true potential when taking exams or attending interviews.
- Difficulties in playing a sport because she becomes needlessly tense and anxious. She may do well when performing in non-competitive situations, but finds it impossible to succeed under pressure.
- Fears about making friends or mixing with other children which result in your child becoming lonely and isolated. Socially anxious youngsters are often regarded as naturally 'shy' and incapable of making many friends. In fact, all children are

naturally sociable and gregarious. They not only enjoy the company of others, but need the stimulation and emotional support that friendships provide.

By teaching your child how to bring anxieties under control you will:

- Increase self-confidence.
- Create a stronger and more positive self-image.
- Ensure greater examination success.
- Improve physical health.
- Help him or her grow into a self-assured adult.
- Provide skills which can be used throughout life for managing stressful situations.

If your child enters adulthood possessing this knowledge he or she will be safeguarded against a wide range of potentially lethal, but entirely avoidable, health problems. These include coronary heart disease, now Western society's number one killer; ulcers; headaches; muscular pains; gastro-intestinal disorders; depression and breakdown.

There is a further benefit from this programme. The easiest way of teaching anxiety-control procedures is to master them yourself first. By doing so you can reduce your own levels of stress, handle situations which now make you unhelpfully anxious with greater ease, and banish any phobias from your life for ever.

Anxiety must be taken seriously

Sadly, many parents treat their child's anxieties far too lightly. They tend to see them either as something that will be outgrown naturally or as a trivial difficulty that could easily be overcome if only the child would make an effort. As a result they respond with either indifference or irritation.

In my experience excessive anxiety is the greatest single threat to successful intellectual, social, emotional, sexual, physical and personal development that any child faces.

Chronic anxiety makes it extremely difficult, often impossible, to understand lessons, solve problems, take decisions, pass exams, do well at interviews, play competitive games, make friends and get along with grown-ups. It also has a devastating long term effect on self-image and self-confidence.

The overly anxious child is timid, unadventurous, and underachieving. He or she has a low self-esteem and a negative self-image. The normal setbacks and upsets of childhood, such as criticism from a teacher, a poor exam result or failure to do as well as expected in some challenge, can overwhelm an already anxious child.

Despite what many parents believe, such anxieties cannot be removed by exhortations to 'stop being stupid', derisive comments about courage or personality, or even sympathetic encouragement and understanding. Trying to jolly a fearful child into a state of calm self-confidence is as futile as attempting to ridicule him into self-assured accomplishment.

Nor do childhood anxieties necessarily vanish of their own accord. While, as we shall see in the next chapter, children do grow out of certain types of anxiety, others will persist into adulthood unless identified and eliminated early.

Martin – a child transformed by anxiety

I first met five-year-old Martin Brown* two weeks before he first went to school. A cheerful and confident little boy, he chatted excitedly about making friends, starting lessons and being as grown-up as his big brother.

Twelve months later, when his worried parents brought him for a consultation, it was hard to recognise Martin as the same enthusiastic, energetic child I had seen just one year earlier.

His whole body was a picture of mental and physical distress. His shoulders drooped, his eyes were downcast and his face a pale mask of unhappiness. All his old energy and enthusiasm was gone, leaving him apathetic and indifferent. His former ebullient self-confidence and bold curiosity had been replaced by a wary uncertainty. He held his mother's hand tightly and clung to her as we chatted.

---

* His name has been changed, as have those of all the other children mentioned in this book.

Mary Brown explained that her son, previously an excellent sleeper, found it hard to get to sleep. And, when he did, his rest was frequently disturbed by terrifying nightmares. His once hearty appetite had disappeared, he took scant interest in his food and ate little. He cried easily, often for no apparent reason, and tired quickly. From being an easy-going child, Martin had developed into a temperamental one who flew into a rage at the slightest provocation. Finally, he was so physically run down that he caught every cold and tummy bug around.

This unhappy transformation was not, however, caused by any physical illness. All the changes I saw were the results of tense and chronic anxiety. At the age of six, he was experiencing the same levels of stress normally suffered by excessively ambitious adults.

For his parents a major barrier to helping Martin was their inability to find out why he had become so anxious. They were sure he wasn't being bullied by other children or badly treated by his teachers. He had always seemed a very bright child, whom they both encouraged to do well. First term reports had described him as of above-average ability and very hard-working.

The key to Martin's anxiety was found to lie in his extreme fear of failure, a common problem which I shall be discussing in greater detail in Chapter Eleven. The boy was so worried about doing well in order to win the approval of adults, especially his rather over-perfectionist parents, that every setback or error in class made him feel guilty, inadequate and at risk of losing their love. Fuelling these fears was the fact that increasing anxiety inevitably led to decreased attainment. The more anxious Martin became over success, the more likely he was to fail.

His anxiety was successfully treated, using the approach described in this book, and the self-fulfilling fear of failure transformed into a strong, positive need for achievement. Now aged eleven, Martin is an emotionally stable, happy youngster, popular with other pupils and well thought of by his teachers. His school work has improved significantly, and mistakes are no longer regarded as a cause for excessive distress.

Now let's look at two other ways in which childhood anxieties can strike.

Sally – a spider phobic

Six months before I started working with Martin, I met a slender, dark-haired nine-year-old named Sally.

Unlike the Browns, Sally's parents knew exactly what caused their daughter's anxiety – she was petrified of spiders. Neither their size or appearance made any difference to the intensity of Sally's fear. Tiny or huge, hairy or hairless, the girl was terrified of them all. Even seeing a spider on television, hearing the word spoken aloud or reading it in a book made her shiver with fear, while seeing a real live one crawling across the floor would send Sally screaming from the room.

At first Sally's parents had treated her fears as something of a joke. Then they tried to reassure her by insisting that there was 'nothing to be frightened of'. Next they became irritated, and accused her of making a fuss over nothing. 'You're too big a girl to be so silly,' they would tell her crossly. 'For goodness sake pull yourself together and act your age!'

Finally, as their daughter's spider phobia started to interfere with her school work, they got worried. This problem began when another child hid a rubber joke-shop spider in her desk. She found it in the middle of a lesson, screamed in horror, burst into tears and fled from the classroom. Sally was so scared that, for a while, she refused to go back into the class at all. Having been persuaded to return, she then refused to open her desk unless the teacher first checked it for spiders.

Sally's terror of spiders was successfully treated by her parents once they had been told what to do and, just as importantly, what *not* to do in order to remove the fear for good. Although she still does not much care for them, Sally is now able to pick them up in a glass and remove them from the room. I shall describe the programme they used, and which you can employ to help your child overcome a phobia, in Chapter Fourteen.

Max – failure from fear

Finally, let me tell you about Max, an athletic fifteen-year-old who, as captain of his school's swimming team, often led them to victory.

Tall, sturdy and self-assured, fair-haired Max seemed the sort of teenager who would fear nothing and no one. Nor did he – with one exception. Exams and tests transformed him from a self-assured young man into a nervous wreck. Even the sight of a question paper caused Max to panic. His stomach churned, his palms sweated; he felt giddy, sick and absolutely convinced that he would never be able to understand, let alone answer, a single question.

It wasn't, however, that Max was idle, unintelligent, or unable to remember what he learned. On the contrary, he was a clever and studious young man with an excellent memory. Yet, judged by exam grades and test scores, he could have been mistaken for the laziest, least capable student in school.

As with Martin and Sally, Max was able to overcome his examination fears by learning some easily mastered skills and applying them to his difficulties.

This book, then, is about the anxieties of young people like Martin, Sally, Max and, perhaps, your own child as well.

Anxiety, fear and phobias

As these case histories show, anxiety can take different forms. Martin's anxiety was all-pervasive and surrounded him like a black cloud from the moment he woke up to the time he fell asleep. Sally and Max's fears were more precisely focused. They knew what caused them and, when not confronting either spiders or exams, were neither perpetually anxious nor persistently unhappy.

So let's consider these three types of emotional response – *general anxiety, fear* and *phobias* – in more detail.

Anxiety

This word is used to describe a state of being troubled by an uncertain, unspecified circumstance – either inside or outside oneself – that threatens some kind of serious harm.

The mental and physical distress involved cannot be linked to any specific person, animal, object, situation, circumstance or activity. The word anxiety – like anger and anguish – is derived from the Latin *angere*: to choke, torment, oppress or cause pain.

You'll find other mental and physical symptoms of anxiety, which are the same as for phobias and fears, listed below. I shall also be describing them in more detail in the next chapter, and explaining what causes them.

Symptoms of anxiety

What goes on in the body
Rapidly beating heart
Dry mouth
Fast breathing
Upset tummy
Need to use lavatory a lot
Sweating
Feeling light-headed or giddy
Going pale or blushing
Trembling hands, tension, headaches, fatigue, loss of appetite

What goes on in the brain
Confused thoughts
Poor memory
Negative thoughts (e.g. 'I can't cope')
Loss of confidence
Panic-filled thoughts
Desire to escape
Poor self-esteem
Bad dreams, night terrors
Silly mistakes are made

Fear
This is anxiety aroused by something your child can see, hear, feel or experience, such as a dog, a loud noise, an injection at the dentist, a stranger.

Your child, when frightened, suffers exactly the same

mental and physical symptoms as when anxious, although they are usually more intense but not so long-lasting. Once the cause of the fear has disappeared the symptoms quickly vanish.

For example, Max experienced great fear in the examination room, yet felt perfectly calm again as soon as the exam was over.

Phobias

These are named after Phobos, the Greek God of fear. Ancient warriors in Greece would paint his horrific features on their shields in an attempt to terrify the enemy. The word phobia itself means 'dread' or 'horror'. Phobias differ from other kinds of fear in three main ways:

1 The fear is intense.
2 The thing that is feared poses no real threat. A child who fears a large and ferocious dog is merely being sensible, but if the same child is terrified to the same extent by a tiny puppy he is a dog phobic, or 'cynophobic'.
3 The fear is sufficiently powerful to cause the child to try and avoid the situation in future. This may mean that the child will run away and refuse to go near the source of his fears, as when Sally refused to return to the classroom. A child with a school phobia may play truant to try and stay at home with a series of minor illnesses.

When the child cannot physically avoid something, she may absent herself mentally by refusing to think about the thing which scares her. A child with a phobia about arithmetic (*arithmophobia*) will escape into fantasy by daydreaming during lessons. This seems like laziness to many teachers, and such students are often punished for not paying attention.

Another type of avoidance is to deal with whatever causes the fear as quickly as possible. This is running away in a different guise. Phobic children are often very impulsive, because rushing headlong into an anxiety-arousing situation means you don't have time to let the fears overwhelm you – rather like taking a flying leap from the top diving-board instead of standing trembling on the edge.

'Getting it over with' is a common phobia- and fear-controlling strategy in both children and adults. In class it can lead clever and capable children to make stupid mistakes. An arithmophobic student, for example, may rush through a maths test in order to complete the painful task as swiftly as possible. This leads to careless errors and easily avoided blunders.

Your child may become phobic about anything. In my time I have seen or treated phobias about blood, vomit, eating in public, going to the lavatory, playing sports, nudity, travelling on a bus or train, pencils, pens, paintbrushes, thunder, insects, cats, dogs, spiders, thunder storms, darkness, horses and hair – to name but a few.

An analysis of more than 2,000 letters received by the charity Action on Phobias, which I established to help phobia-sufferers, is shown below. The percentage of sufferers – mainly adults – with each type of phobia is also given.

As the table shows, the most common problem is agoraphobia. This is not, as many believe, a fear of open spaces, but of going into public places such as crowded streets or busy stores. Like the name for most phobias it comes from a Greek word, *agora*, meaning a place where people gather.

Type of Phobia	% Presenting	Number	Rank
Acne	0.08	2	31
Acrophobia	2.02	49	9
Agoraphobia	36.78	893	1
Androphobia	0.16	4	29
Anything decapitated	0.04	1	32
Anything large	0.04	1	32
Anything squashed	0.04	1	32
Asbestos	0.04	1	32
Babies and children	0.12	3	30
Bees and wasps	1.07	26	13
Being alone	1.11	27	12
Being attacked	0.08	2	31
Being away from home	0.12	3	30
Being driven by car	1.77	43	9
Birds	1.77	43	9
Blood	0.49	12	22

Type of Phobia	% Presenting	Number	Rank
Blushing	0.78	19	17
Body odour	0.37	9	25
Bridges	0.82	20	16
Breath stopping	0.16	4	29
Buried alive	0.20	5	28
Butterflies and moths	1.02	25	14
Buttons	0.08	2	31
Cats	0.66	16	18
Chickens	0.08	2	31
Cooking	0.58	14	20
Claustrophobia	7.04	171	2
Cobwebs	0.04	1	32
Coiled springs	0.04	1	32
Cows	0.04	1	32
Crowds	0.91	22	15
Darkness	0.25	6	27
Dead animals	0.04	1	32
Death	1.89	46	8
Dirt and germs	0.54	13	21
Dogs	1.56	38	10
Driving a car	0.62	15	19
Dusk	0.04	1	32
Eating in public	1.52	37	11
Escalators	0.12	3	30
Faeces	0.04	1	32
Fainting	0.45	11	23
Falling	0.25	6	27
Feathers	0.49	12	22
Fires	0.04	1	32
Flying	3.21	78	6
Footballs	0.04	1	32
Frogs	0.12	3	30
Fumes	0.04	1	32
Gasholders	0.04	1	32
God	0.08	2	31
Hair loss	0.08	2	31
Hard surfaces	0.08	2	31
Harming people	0.20	5	28
Hedgehogs	0.04	1	32
Hell and the devil	0.04	1	32
High buildings	0.62	15	19

Type of Phobia	% Presenting	Number	Rank
Hills	0.16	4	29
Holidays	0.37	9	25
Horses	0.20	5	28
Hospitals	0.12	3	30
Ice and snow	0.12	3	30
Illness	1.77	43	9
Injections	0.41	10	24
Insects	0.41	10	24
Kenophobia	0.08	2	31
Kerbs	0.04	1	32
Lifts	0.16	4	29
Loud noises	0.62	15	19
Mirrors	0.04	1	32
Monkeys	0.04	1	32
Needing lavatory	0.29	7	26
Nudity	0.08	2	31
Old age	0.04	1	32
Oral exams	0.08	2	31
Own thoughts	0.16	4	26
People	4.00	97	3
Plants and undergrowth	0.04	1	32
Pregnancy	0.04	1	32
Public speaking	0.16	4	26
Public transport	3.21	78	5
Rats and mice	0.66	16	18
Sex	0.25	6	27
Sleep	0.25	6	27
Snails	0.04	1	32
Snakes	0.41	10	24
Spiders	2.84	69	6
Steps	0.08	2	31
Sweating	0.04	1	32
Telephones	0.20	5	25
Thunder	6.34	154	3
Vomit	3.46	84	5
Water	0.41	10	24
Whales	0.04	1	32
Wide roads	0.16	4	29
Windy weather	0.37	9	25
Worms	0.20	5	28
Writing in public	0.16	4	29

With the exception of agoraphobia, which may start in the teens but more usually develops during the early twenties, all the phobias listed can afflict children as badly as adults. How and why these fears, many of which may strike you as bizarre, arise I shall explain later in the book.

The most tragic case I have ever encountered was an eleven-year-old boy who had become phobic about his mother. This started when the child was three. Although not absolutely certain what had caused it, his mother believed the fears first started when some clothes she had washed for him became accidentally infested with bugs. From then on his fear of her grew progressively worse. He refused to eat the food she prepared or wear any clothes she laundered. Eventually he could not even stay in the same house and moved in with his grandmother, who lived nearby. If his mother attempted to hold or cuddle him, he screamed and struggled to get away. On one occasion, his mother told me she had said to him sadly: 'I know you can never love me, darling, but couldn't we even be friends?'

As he grew older the fears were somewhat reduced, but even into his teens they made it impossible for him to enjoy a normal, loving relationship with his mother.

This was a very unusual case, and one where the fear had lasted so long, and was so intense, that professional assistance was essential in order to resolve it – and even then with only partial success. Few phobias are so complex and intractable, however. In the vast majority of cases you are perfectly capable of teaching your child the procedures needed to overcome his or her anxieties, fears and phobias.

To do so you must:

Understand anxiety

Most people know what it feels like to be anxious. Many, if not all, the symptoms listed in Box One will be familiar to almost every reader. But have you ever wondered why we should have to suffer such disagreeable and, seemingly, damaging thoughts and feelings?

Knowing why anxiety arises and produces these unpleasant mental and physical symptoms is the first step towards its conquest. An understanding of the underlying bodily mechanisms, and their important biological purpose, helps make them less frightening and easier to bring under control.

Appreciating what's happening inside your child's body when he or she becomes anxious, fearful or phobic is going to help you approach the task of eliminating those negative feelings more expertly and confidently. I shall explain the bodily mechanisms responsible for feelings of anxiety in the next chapter.

Know why your child becomes anxious

Clearly, until the cause or causes have been pinpointed little can be done to bring them under control. Only after they had discovered why their son was so unhappy could Martin's parents set about first reducing, and finally removing, his anxieties.

Sometimes the reasons for your child's difficulties are either obvious, or not hard to discover. This is especially true about so-called monophobias, where there is a single object, animal, activity, etc. which triggers the fears.

On other occasions the cause of the fear may seem obvious, but actually prove quite hard to track down. Suppose, for instance, your child is apprehensive and pleads for a sick-note on games afternoons. It is clearly that something to do with playing sport is triggering his anxiety. However, this still leaves a wide range of possibilities open.

Perhaps he is scared of being injured during a rough game. Maybe he is fearful of bullying classmates or a sarcastic PE master. He could be fearful of letting his side down by playing badly, or of making a mistake and being ridiculed by the other boys. In some schools, team captains select their sides from a group of children, naturally choosing the best players first and then selecting, with obvious reluctance, from the less athletic and physically weaker youngsters who remain. The humiliation of being chosen last, and then with obvious displeasure, may be sufficiently traumatic to produce chronic anxiety in a sensitive child.

The fears might, equally, have nothing to do with the

games themselves but focus on changing-room behaviour. Public undressing, and the communal nudity of compulsory showers or baths, can greatly upset some children, especially around puberty. Sexual horseplay in the changing-rooms is another possible cause of anxiety and distress.

As you can see, even when you know where to search for clues, identifying the source of anxiety is not always straightforward or easy. And it is often hard even to know where to start looking. Young children often lack the words needed to express their fears, while older ones may be embarrassed or concerned that their admissions will make you think badly of them.

I shall be explaining how to pinpoint the source of anxieties in Chapter Seven.

Create your child's personal training plan

Because each child differs from every other in terms of personality, attitudes, experiences and outlook on life, there can never be a rigidly defined approach to the treatment of anxiety. There are certain basic procedures of well-proven clinical value, but these can be worse than useless when applied insensitively or without adequate thought.

The challenge you face is to create a training programme tailored to meet your child's unique individual needs. If this sounds rather daunting, please do not feel discouraged. In my experience, not only do most parents master the procedures with ease, but they find working with their child to remove handicapping anxieties immensely reassuring and rewarding.

There can be few more satisfying experiences for a loving parent than to see a once-frightened child become smiling and confident as anxious self-doubt is replaced by certainty and self-confidence.

Two

Your Questions Answered

I am sure there would be many questions you would like to ask if we were able to chat about your child's anxieties. Although I cannot, of course, know exactly what specific queries or concern you might have, experience suggests that one or more of the following would be on your list.

Question One: How can I tell whether my child has an anxiety problem?

This is a question which we shall be exploring in more detail in later chapters.

Anxiety often makes its presence felt in a disguised form. As a result it tends to get dismissed as laziness, stupidity, lack of nerve or loss of confidence. Or it can express itself as an illness; although the underlying cause is emotional rather than physical, these ailments are perfectly genuine with real symptoms like tummy upsets, muscle cramps and headaches. Anxiety may be mistaken for growing pains, jealousy, bad temper, hyperactivity, impulsiveness, aggression and many other types of behaviour not usually considered to have anything to do with being anxious, fearful or phobic.

In Chapter Three I will be explaining in detail how you can explore your child's anxieties and identify likely causes. Here's a quick check to help you decide whether your child is suffering from too much anxiety.

All you have to do is note the statements which best

describe your child's behaviour over the past six months. I suggest that you then repeat the procedure to assess your own levels of anxiety.

My child:

1 sleeps badly (i.e. finds it hard to drop off or wakes often): a: seldom or never; b: occasionally; c: all the time.

2 has a poor appetite: a: seldom or never; b: occasionally; c: all the time.

3 becomes very irritable over minor setbacks: a: seldom or never; b: occasionally; c: all the time.

4 cries for no apparent reason: a: seldom or never; b: occasionally; c: all the time.

5 has many minor illnesses (e.g. colds, tummy upsets) a: seldom or never; b: occasionally; c: all the time.

6 is sullen and moody: a: seldom or never; b: occasionally; c: all the time.

7 is reluctant to attempt new challenges: a: seldom or never; b: occasionally; c: all the time.

8 behaviour is disruptive at home or school: a: seldom or never; b: occasionally; c: all the time.

9 has fallen behind in class for no apparent reason: a: not at all; b: to some extent; c: very much so.

10 has started wetting the bed again: a: seldom or never; b: occasionally; c: all the time.

11 becomes tired very easily: a: seldom or never; b: occasionally; c: all the time.

12 is fearful when attempting anything new: a: seldom or never; b: occasionally; c: all the time.

13 gets very upset over justifiable criticisms: a: seldom or never; b: occasionally; c: all the time.

14 is shy about meeting others: a: seldom or never; b: occasionally; c: all the time.

15 dislikes staying with friends or relatives: a: seldom or never; b: occasionally; c: all the time.

16 finds it hard to make friends: a: seldom or never; b: occasionally; c: all the time.

17 asks to be excused school on certain days: a: seldom or never; b: occasionally; c: frequently.

18 has nightmares: a: seldom or never; b: occasionally; c: frequently.

19 dislikes changes in routine: **a**: seldom or never; **b**: occasionally; **c**: all the time.
20 finds it hard to stand up for himself or herself: **a**: seldom or never; **b**: occasionally; **c**: all the time.

If testing yourself, or a child older than thirteen, change statements 8, 9, 10, 14, 15, 17 as follows:

8 I am restless and find it hard to stay still: **a**: seldom or never; **b**: occasionally; **c**: all the time.
9 I find it as easy to do the things I used to do: **a**: very much so; **b**: to some extent; **c**: not at all.
10 I feel tense or wound up: **a**: seldom or never; **b**: occasionally; **c**: all the time.
14 I find it hard to make friends: **a**: seldom or never; **b**: occasionally; **c**: all the time.
15 I get anxious when invited to a party: **a**: seldom or never; **b**: occasionally; **c**: all the time.
17 I avoid certain tasks or activities: **a**: seldom or never; **b**: occasionally; **c**: all the time.

How to score

Award 5 points for each **c**, 2 for each **b** and 0 for each **a**. This gives a possible maximum score of 100.

Score range	Likely anxiety levels
0–25	Unlikely to be any chronic anxiety problem, although he/she may still be made anxious by specific activities or events.
26–40	A low level of general anxiety which may lead to occasional problems.
41–60	A moderate level of general anxiety. It may be making itself felt in moodiness, bursts of irritation or a reluctance to try anything new.
61–80	A fairly high level of anxiety which could be disrupting your child's life in many different ways, although you may not

always have realised that anxious feelings
were responsible.

80 plus   Your child seems extremely anxious and
unhappy. This will be making life very hard
for him/her in many different ways. Start
work right away to reduce this very high level
of anxiety.

This short assessment is intended to provide only a general
indication of whether or not your child is being restricted by
harmfully high levels of anxiety. Any score above 25 suggests
that you would be well advised to study and use the
procedures for managing anxiety described in this book.

You should also take into account your own level of
anxiety. If you obtained a score higher than 20, while your
child does not appear to be excessively anxious, I suggest
you use the plan described in Chapter Ten to reduce your
own level of anxiety. This will help prevent your feelings
from increasing your child's anxieties (see Question Two).
The same applies if you both obtained scores greater than
20.

Question Two: Can my child 'catch' anxiety from me?

This is a question I am often asked, frequently by mothers
who are phobic themselves. They worry that their intense
fears will be passed on to their child. Well, in the sense that
you might pass on a cold germ or flu virus, the answer is
obviously no. There are, however, two ways in which
parental anxieties can be communicated to their children.
The first is through their genes, the second through the way
they behave.

As we shall see later in the book, babies are not born with
specific fears. If you are a very agoraphobic mother, for
example, your infant is not going to be born pre-programmed
with agoraphobia. But what does tend to happen is that a
tendency towards anxiety, a vulnerability to fears and
phobias, can run in the family – in the same way that if you
breed from two very nervous cats, their kittens are more

likely than average to have a nervous disposition. This doesn't mean for certain that all, or even any of them, must inevitably be anxious. It just increases the chances.

Many years ago Dr Hans Eysenck demonstrated that an important difference between extroverts and introverts lies in the way in which their nervous systems function. Extroverts, with their love of bustle, noise and excitement, tend to have nervous systems which demand a great deal of stimulation to be fully activated. Introverts, with their desire for a quiet life, require far less stimulation in order to feel pleasantly aroused. A level of excitement which an extrovert would find comfortably stimulating could drive an introvert to distraction. It is the same with anxiety. Situations which one person can cope with easily will make another extremely anxious.

The second way in which anxieties can be passed on is by teaching your child through example. If you are terrified of spiders, for instance, your child may acquire the same fear just by watching you in action.

In both cases, however, there is much that can be done to bring anxiety under control. Even children who possess high levels of what is termed 'trait' anxiety, i.e. an inborn tendency to feel anxious, can be taught ways of controlling their mental and physical responses.

Question Three: How unusual are anxiety problems?

Anxiety and fears are facts of life for even the most secure and well-cared-for child. In one of the earliest studies, carried out in 1934 by Arthur T. Jerslid and F.B. Holmes, childhood fears were reported by virtually all the parents questioned. Later research confirmed this finding, with 90 per cent of mothers admitting that their child suffered at least one specific fear at some time between the ages of two and fourteen years.

Question Four: Why is my child scared of so many things?

There is nothing unusual in a child being frightened of several things. In fact, research has shown that the majority of children suffer from more than one fear or anxiety. An American study of nearly 500 children aged between six and twelve revealed that 43 per cent had more than seven fears of one sort or another.

Question Five: Which fears are most common?

This varies according to your child's age. What terrifies a toddler may leave an eight-year-old completely unconcerned. Many infants, for instance, are wary of strangers and hate being separated from their parents – especially their mother. By the age of three or four, these fears have usually been replaced by anxieties about monsters or ghosts.

Older children are made anxious by the idea of physical injury, classroom failure or not living up to their parents' expectations. Eight out of ten five- and six-year-olds admitted to being fearful of animals, while only two out of ten thirteen- and fourteen-year-olds did so. Fears of ghosts, common among nursery-school children, have generally gone for good by the age of ten.

As children get into their teens, anxieties about the future, and the way it will affect their lives, tend to predominate. A

What makes your child afraid	
Age	Main fears
0–2	Loud noises. Strange objects, people and situations. Falling. Separation from parents.
2–4	Sudden movement, flashing lights, shadows. Animals. Scary dreams.
4–6	Ghosts, darkness, imaginary creatures, dreams, death, robbers.
6 onwards	Being teased, scolded, punished, criticised, reprimanded or feeling humiliated. Loss of love or respect of parents, physical pain, natural events (e.g. storms), relations with other children, school, exams, sports, nudity (e.g. showers, changing rooms), sex.

recent study of teenagers by Pam Gillies, a lecturer in community health at the University of Nottingham Medical School, revealed fears about unemployment (mentioned by 81 per cent), poverty (52 per cent) and nuclear war (33 per cent). AIDS was mentioned by nearly a sixth of the fifteen- to sixteen-year-olds she questioned. Other significant anxieties included the dangers of childbirth and the risk of marriage ending in divorce; sexual anxieties and fear of physical injury are also common.

Early fears – such as of spooks and ghouls, witches and monsters – are likely to be the result of a vivid but imperfectly controlled imagination. As your child learns more about the world, and gains greater control over his or her fantasies, imaginary fears give way to more realistic ones, such as concern with injury, physical danger, school achievements, competing in sports and games, making friends with other children, being bullied or being excluded from groups.

Question Six: Will my child just grow out of his or her fears?

While anxieties, fears and phobias are more likely to disappear of their own accord in children than in adults, time is often an unreliable healer.

When researchers looked at the fears of ten-year-olds over a twelve-month period, for instance, they found little change in either the number or the type reported. What's more, fears which develop from around the age of eleven onwards often continue into adult life. The child who is afraid of strangers may well grow up into a shy, perhaps rather lonely, adult. The youngster who has a deep-rooted dread of failure is likely to develop into an overly cautious grown-up with poor self-esteem and little ambition.

Anxiety takes its toll in another way, too. However clever and capable they are, overly anxious students will never do as well as those who can remain calm and confident when confronting intellectual challenges. No matter what your child is attempting, from doing sums to writing an essay, from speaking in class to painting in art, excessive anxiety makes failure more likely than success. This means that the anxious child never realizes his or her true intellectual potential. Class marks are poor, examination grades low. And the highly competitive nature of today's job market makes it increasingly hard to recover from such early setbacks.

For all these reasons it is essential to take your child's anxieties and fears seriously – not only to alleviate needless suffering and distress in the short term, but to prevent avoidable, long-term emotional, social and intellectual damage.

Question Seven: If I help remove one fear, won't another take its place?

No. This hardly ever happens. Freud believed that fears like Sally's terror of spiders are merely symptoms of a far deeper problem. However, most modern clinicians agree that if you take away a fear nothing else takes place. To use a piece of therapy jargon, there is no 'symptom substitution'. In other words, when Sally's spider phobia was removed she did not suddenly become phobic about mice or cats or thunderstorms.

Question Eight: When should I seek professional help?

There are some anxiety problems which do require professional help on a one-to-one basis. These include the more complicated and chronic conditions, where anxiety difficulties have been allowed to build up over a long period of time. Occasionally, too, a child may suffer a single but severely traumatic experience, such as an indecent assault, where the experience and knowledge of a trained therapist will be needed to repair the damage.

The importance of parent power

There are three reasons why parents are usually in the best possible position to help their children.

Firstly, who knows your child better than you do? Who

else can observe changing moods and activity on an hour-by-hour, day-to-day basis? Your unique knowledge means that you can create a plan tailored precisely to your child's individual needs, and then implement it in the way most likely to bring about beneficial change.

Secondly, a child's anxiety often reflects stresses and tensions within the family as a whole. This doesn't mean that an anxious child must always be the victim of a miserable marriage or an unhappy home. While such problems can certainly trigger and sustain these difficulties, childhood anxieties are just as often found in youngsters from happy and loving families. None the less, it is useful to consider how your own attitudes and outlook on life, as well as those of your partner and other children in the family, may be influencing an overly anxious child's approach to living.

Finally, your child can learn to overcome his or her fears and anxieties most easily in the security of a warm and reassuring family environment.

In the next chapter we shall be taking our first step towards creating such a training programme, by finding out what causes anxieties and how they can best be overcome.

Three
Why Your Child Gets Anxious

While you are shopping in the busy high street, your five-year-old wanders away. The next second you spot her about to dash from behind a parked car into the path of an oncoming bus.

Your terrified response to this situation will involve many of the symptoms described on page 10. Your heart races, your stomach turns over, your mouth goes dry. You call urgently and, thankfully, your child hurries back. The shock of that near tragedy leaves you feeling sick, shaking and faint.

Great anxiety, as anybody who has ever been acutely anxious well knows, is extremely handicapping. No one can think clearly or act decisively when their body is racked by painful symptoms and their mind confused by fearful thoughts. So why should anything as seemingly unnecessary, unhelpful and uncomfortable as the anxiety response have evolved? What possible purpose can it serve?

By understanding the nature and function of anxiety you'll be able to help your child, and yourself, deal with it more positively and effectively.

Fighting or fleeing

Imagine that you turn the corner in your high street and come face to face with an escaped circus lion – what would you do?

Apart from allowing yourself to be eaten, there are only two choices – fight or flee. In order to do either successfully your body must swiftly become aroused. Your heart will have to beat faster, to speed oxygen-rich blood to brain and muscles, so your pulse rate increases from around 65 beats per minute to 180 or more. You breathe more rapidly to take in extra oxygen and expel the large amounts of potentially lethal carbon dioxide produced by vigorous action. As a result your chest feels tight and you may start panting.

The blood is diverted away from the muscles of throat, stomach and digestive tract, and from tiny vessels (capillaries) directly beneath the skin, in order to make more available for the arms and legs. Your digestion slows, your mouth goes dry, your stomach feels queasy, you grow pale.

The muscles in your arms, legs, shoulders and back tense in preparation for vigorous action. This tension can make you tremble at the time, and feel cramped, sore and painful once the emergency is over.

Oxygen-laden blood sent to the brain helps you think quickly and have lightning-fast reactions, but this can also leave you feeling light-headed, giddy or faint. You may also experience problems with your balance or vision. The ground could suddenly seem to sway under your feet. Walls, hedges and fences may appear to be falling away or about to collapse on top of you. There is often a sense of unreality, a feeling that everything is happening in a dream and that you no longer have any existence as an individual.

As you fight or flee, the vigorous action produces a great deal of heat. To keep cool you'll sweat profusely. This lowers your temperature as it evaporates from the skin. Your fear can also lead to a drop in body temperature as blood is diverted away from the capillaries just beneath the skin. To combat this loss, your body will attempt to erect hairs which our ape ancestors had in such abundance. Today all we can manage is goose pimples, although those hairs we do have may stand on end!

If there really were a lion on the loose, or some other genuine threat to life and limb, all these changes – far from being useless and unnecessary – could ensure your survival. Suddenly you'll possess strength, stamina and endurance which, in your normal unaroused state, you would never experience.

An excellent illustration of our body's untapped physical prowess is to be found in the remarkable story of Dr Murray Watson's bush shorts.

The case of the torn bush shorts

Although they are old and minus a seat, zoologist Murray Watson cherishes a pair of bush shorts as a souvenir of his one death-defying leap. It happened while he was studying elephants in Kenya's Tsavo National Park and his Land-rover broke down on the way back to camp, one moonless evening, leaving him with the choice of spending a shivering night in the cab or walking a short distance to a comfortable bed.

Despite the danger from wild animals, 26-year-old Murray Watson immediately started back for his camp. He had only gone a few hundred feet from the vehicle when he realised that this was probably the worst decision of his life. As he stumbled along the dirt track in almost complete darkness, Murray heard the sound of grunts and padding feet close behind him.

Shortly before the Land-Rover's engine stalled he had seen a hyena pack feeding on carrion in the twilight. Now he knew they were following him. The young zoologist started running, but it was too late. The hyenas closed for the kill. A tree suddenly loomed up out of the darkness and Murray Watson took a flying leap for the lowest branch. As he swung himself to safety the pack leader's teeth shredded the seat of his pants. Murray spent an uncomfortable night clinging to the branch, with the hyena pack waiting below.

It was full daylight before they reluctantly abandoned their vigil and slunk away into the bush. Only then, as he attempted to clamber down from his branch, did Murray Watson realise just how remarkable his escape had been. The branch that had saved his life was a good twelve feet above the ground. Once he had climbed down there was no way he could get back up again. His best leap for the branch fell at least four feet short.

Murray Watson's torn bush shorts are a potent reminder of his one and only Olympic gold-medal leap. A tribute not to any athletic ability but to the latent power of the human body – a power which it often takes acute anxiety to release.

There are two key points to note about this switch from a very relaxed to a highly aroused state: it's fast and it's automatic.

Why the switch is fast

As they scavenged warily across the open savannah, the forebears of modern man had to respond instantly to the slightest evidence of such ferocious predators as sabretooth tigers, lions and leopards.

A movement, half glimpsed through the undergrowth, the rustle of leaves or the snap of a twig could all warn of imminent danger. Under those conditions speed of arousal was crucial. Any time lost debating whether the threat was a real or imagined one could mean the difference between living and dying. Today, millions of years later, our ability to become instantly aroused is a legacy of our ancestors' precarious lifestyle.

Why the switch is automatic

When survival demands fast reactions rather than intellectual reflection, the sensible thing to do is fight or flee first and ask questions later. For this, and other life-sustaining purposes, a separate nervous system has evolved. This independent mechanism, whose activities are not under the direct control of our 'thinking brain' is called the autonomic nervous system, usually abbreviated to ANS. Among the ANS's daily concerns are keeping the heart beating, digesting food, maintaining body temperature and regulating breathing. Without these vital, but routine, functions being fully automated life would be impossible. Imagine trying to get your children off to school, while digesting your breakfast, telling your heart to beat once a second, instructing your lungs to fill 800 times an hour, keeping your body at a steady 98.4°F., monitoring blood pressure and so on.

The ANS is also in charge of arousing the body when under threat. But because it is not under voluntary control, our 'thinking brain' is unable to prevent this arousal. Even when we know there is no danger, we'll still become anxious if the ANS commands us to.

This poses problems. Imagine the human pilot of an aircraft locked on automatic pilot attempting to prevent a crash course by chatting politely to the computer. As a wall of mountain looms up in the cockpit window, he suggests that the robot gain altitude or take some other avoiding action. The computer, naturally, takes no notice and continues to fly according to its previously programmed instructions. It's the same with our built-in auto pilot, the ANS, whenever we try to change its actions by conscious thought.

You cannot, for instance, stop your stomach digesting food or your heart pumping blood by telling them to do so. Sally, whose terror of spiders I described in Chapter One, knew perfectly well that her fear was irrational, but that didn't make it any the less terrifying. Max recognised that his intense anxiety over examinations was unnecessary and self-destructive, but this made not the slightest difference to the way he felt or responded.

For reasons which we will examine below, their automatic pilots had learned to see these situations as a genuine threat, and that was how they responded.

Speed-up, slow-down

To see exactly how anxiety arises, we need to explore the ANS in more detail. The system has two branches. One speeds things up, and is responsible for arousal, while the other slows them down again. Their different effects on the way your body works are summarized below.

Step-up		Slow-down
Increased	Heart rate	Decreased
Decreased	Digestion	Increased
Increased	Muscle tension	Decreased
Decreased	Blood to stomach and gut	Increased
Increased	Blood to muscles	Decreased

Decreased	Blood to skin	Increased
Increased	Blood pressure	Decreased
Increased	Sweating	Decreased
Decreased	Energy reserves	Increased
Increased	Oxygen used	Decreased

Although their effects on the body are entirely different, these two branches normally co-operate to keep everything working smoothly. They can be likened to the reins of a horse. When the rider uses equal pressure on each rein the horse goes in a straight line. But if greater force is applied to one side the horse turns in that direction.

While the *slow-down* branch is in control you feel calm and relaxed. Your blood pressure and heart rate are slowed, breathing is light, food is digested, your muscles relax.

As the *step-up* branch takes charge, which it does whenever danger seems to threaten, the exact opposite occurs. Heart rate and blood pressure increase, your digestion may be disturbed, you perspire more freely. The output of an important stress-related substance called corticosteroid, produced by the adrenal glands above each kidney, increases.

These changes are brought about by the actions of chemical messengers which are pumped into the blood at the command of the ANS and circulate rapidly around the entire body. The best known of these, adrenaline (known in the US as epinephrine) is sometimes dubbed 'jungle juice' because of its central role in the fight or flight response.

The sensation of unease in the pit of your stomach, which is so often the forerunner of anxiety, is due to the hormone adrenaline pouring into the blood stream at the command of the ANS's step-up branch.

Your child and the ANS

To get a clearer picture of how all this would affect your child's physical and mental state, let's imagine that he is very afraid of the class bully. This older, bigger boy has threatened to beat him up after school.

As he starts for home, in the evening twilight, your child is already apprehensive. His heart is beating slightly faster than usual, and his stomach feels queasy. Turning into a deserted street, he catches a glimpse of a boy who looks like the bully emerging from an alley some distance ahead.

While the 'thinking' part of your child's mind is trying to decide whether the figure really is his sworn enemy or not, the step-up branch of his ANS has swung into instant action.

His heart pounds, he trembles and feels sick, his mouth is suddenly dry and he breathes rapidly and unevenly. Just as he is wondering whether to turn and run or confront the bully, the person walks under a street lamp and is recognised as his best friend. There is an immediate feeling of relief. The slow-down mechanism takes over and, gradually, your child's heart stops racing and his breathing becomes regular again.

But suppose it had been the bully, intent on carrying out his threat. Your child would turn and run flat out for the safety of a crowded shopping mall. With the danger passed, his slow-down mechanism can again restore his body to normal running.

Similarly, if he had decided to confront and fight the bully, the energy used up in the struggle would have made it easier for his slow-down branch to bring things under control once the struggle was over. In both these cases, of course, his arousal served a helpful purpose.

However, the fear created by seeing a possible attacker emerge from that alley could also have serious longer-term consequences for your son. We'll imagine that there was no bully. The threat was an empty one. He is never in any real danger. None the less, the fear he felt as the unidentified youngster emerged suddenly from the alley might become linked in his mind with that street, or with any street which has side turnings similar to the alley.

The next time he walks home from school your son might decide to take a slightly longer route home because it keeps him away from the street. After a while he finds it impossible to walk down that particular street, or even similar streets. He would then have become phobic about them. This is a topic I shall be returning to in the final chapter.

For the moment, bear in mind that a bad fright can create a long-term anxiety difficulty through simple association.

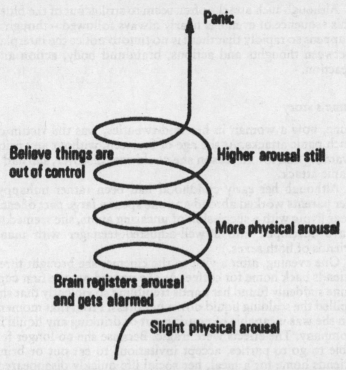

Panic

Believe things are out of control

Higher arousal still

More physical arousal

Brain registers arousal and gets alarmed

Slight physical arousal

So far we have focused on the bodily symptoms of anxiety. But of course physical responses are almost always accompanied by fearful thoughts. The sequence of events is along these lines. Your child is startled. Her attention is drawn to something which, rightly or wrongly, she sees as posing a threat. Negative thoughts pop into her mind. 'I don't like this . . . I shan't be able to cope . . . I am going to make a fool of myself . . . I must get away . . .'

These thoughts feed back into the system and increase the power of the step-up mechanism. The heart starts to beat faster, breathing becomes more rapid. These bodily changes provoke even more desperate and unhelpful thoughts. In turn the mental distress triggers further physical arousal. Within seconds a panic attack can have engulfed the child, as shown in the diagram above.

Although such attacks often seem to strike 'out of the blue', this sequence of events is nearly always followed – though it happens so rapidly that there is no time to notice the interplay between thoughts and actions, brain and body, action and reaction.

June's story

June, now a woman in her mid-twenties, was the victim of such panic attacks. At the age of fourteen, without any prior warning and for no reason she could ever discover, she had a panic attack.

Although her early childhood had been rather unhappy, her parents worked abroad and she spent a large part of each year living with a succession of uncaring aunts, she seemed to have developed into a well-adjusted teenager with many friends of both sexes.

One evening, after a visit to the cinema, she brought three friends back home for coffee. As she poured out the first cup, June suddenly found her hands trembling so violently that she spilled the scalding liquid down her dress. From that moment on she was incapable of pouring out or drinking any liquid in company. The effects were tragic. Because she no longer felt able to go to parties, accept invitations to eat out or bring friends home for a meal, her social life quickly disappeared, leaving her lonely and depressed.

June had been especially keen on science, but now chemistry practicals became a nightmare. Each time she attempted to pour fluids they ended up all over the laboratory bench or floor. She managed to get through the course with the help of a friend who handled all the equipment. Then the trouble spread to her handwriting, which became illegible whenever she was being watched while writing.

Not surprisingly, this undermined her confidence and self-esteem to such an extent that she ended up with examination grades far below her true abilities. As with most anxious students, June never received any sympathy or understanding for her problems. She was criticised by teachers for being clumsy or lazy, for not concentrating, trying or working hard enough. They failed to appreciate the devastating effects of chronic anxiety on her classroom performance. Indeed, the powerful influence of emotions on studying is still largely disregarded in school and colleges. (The Chinese, more perceptively, use a symbol for intelligence made up from icons for both head and heart, thus acknowledging the potent effect that feelings exert over intellectual achievement.)

Old brain and new brain

The human brain is like an immensely ancient house on to which successive generations have added new floors and additional wings. The earliest and most primitive parts (sometimes called the reptilian brain), which are responsible for emotional responses, evolved millions of years before the latest addition – the intellectual powerhouse of the cerebral cortex. This emerged only about 40,000 years ago, hardly a single tick on the evolutionary clock. This means that twentieth-century humans, young and old, are trying to function with emotional machinery better suited to an era when the toxodont, camelid and mastodon roamed the earth.

Survival in the age of information technology seldom requires either fight or flight in the literal sense. Typically, we must cope with threats not to our physical survival but to our emotional or intellectual well-being.

Many children, for instance, become anxious when having to answer questions in front of a class, while being watched in their work by a critical teacher, when being scolded by their parents or while facing a sarcastic grown-up. They suffer acute anxiety when making friends, when teased, mocked or ridiculed by other children. Their level of arousal may soar while revising for, or taking, an exam or being interviewed. Rejection, or the feeling that they have been rejected, can also trigger excessive anxiety.

Despite the fact that none of these situations places them in any real danger, their ANS responds as if they were under physical attack. In the short term, no matter what you are attempting to do, excessive anxiety ensures that you will do it

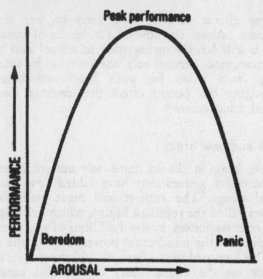

worse. But, paradoxically, when just the right amount of arousal is present we are not handicapped but helped by this low level of anxiety. In fact, we probably don't even interpret the slight rise in heart rate, more rapid breathing and general increase in tension as painful but pleasurable. It helps us perform more efficiently and enjoy life more.

Anxiety can help your child

Dr Hans Selye, a pioneer of stress research, uses the term *eustress* to distinguish controlled and beneficial anxiety levels from the harmful stress which damages performance.

Distress occurs when brain and body are taxed beyond their capacity. This may occur because your child is trying to cope with too many challenges, mental and/or physical, at the same time. But, equally, it can be caused by a lack of stress. Understress, which is usually caused by having to do tedious or routine chores, causes as much harm to health and motivation as overstress. This is the kind of stress problem one finds in very gifted children compelled to follow a school timetable which makes no real demands on their minds.

The relationship between arousal and performance is shown opposite. As you can see, up to a certain point you get better the more aroused your ANS becomes. But, beyond a critical point, performance declines sharply.

Every child, and adult, has a Peak Performance Stress Level (PPSL) which varies between one person and another, and from task to task. For some activities your child needs to become more mentally and physically aroused than for others. But if obliged to work above or below his or her PPSL for more than a short time, performance suffers.

As stress levels rise your child becomes increasingly confused, anxious and uncertain of his or her ability to cope with the demands being made. Memory and concentration falter, so that even well-learned facts and figures are forgotten or inaccurately recalled.

When understressed your child is bored, apathetic, and lacking in motivation. He or she may feel depressed, have a poor appetite and sleep badly, despite feeling tired much of the time. It becomes so hard to make a decision or solve a problem that even simple choices or minor challenges seem impossible.

We can compare our resistance to stress with a bank account. The more we spend, the less we have in reserve to tide us over a rainy day. These savings are regularly renewed by sleeping, eating and relaxation.

Let's imagine that your child has 100 units of stress resistance in her psychological savings bank. Exams are approaching and she is worried about doing badly and letting you down. This anxiety costs her, let's imagine, 40 stress resistance units each day. However, there is no real problem because she still has 60 units in reserve. Each night's rest tops her reserves up again.

Now let's tax her reserves still further by adding some more stressors. She has a row with her best friend. This uses 30 units a day for a week, until the row is settled. She's down to 30 units a day to cope with all the rest of life's stressful events. One day she does some careless work and gets into a row from her teacher. This uses 40 units and causes her to overdraw.

If she only goes into the red occasionally, not much harm

will be done. On those days when she is overdrawn, you'll notice that she's far edgier and more irritable than usual. Depending on her ways of coping with excessive stress, she may fly off the handle or withdraw into a sulk. She'll find it hard to concentrate and perhaps become weepy. But after a night's rest she'll be restored to her former, cheerful and capable self.

If she becomes constantly overdrawn, however, no immediate recovery will be possible. A downward spiral may develop, as she starts eating and sleeping less well, so weakening her resistance. Because psychological stress causes her body's natural defence mechanism, the immune system, to work less efficiently, she runs a greater risk of catching a cold or flu. Fighting these germs will make further demands on her reserves, thus deepening the crisis.

There are certain periods of life, and events in life, which place your child at particularly grave risk from getting into a situation when chronic overdrawing becomes a way of life. The four periods of your child's life when stress is likely to be at its greatest are:

1 Starting school, and making that big change from being with you all day to adjusting to a new routine.
2 Changing schools, and having to make friends – especially the move from primary to secondary education.
3 In the fifth year of secondary education while revising for exams.
4 Around puberty, when mind and body are coming to terms with different ways of feeling and responding.

The six most stressful life events a child may have to cope with are:

1 The death of a relative or close friend.
2 The break-up of your marriage.
3 Father being made redundant.
4 Moving home.
5 The death of a much-loved pet.
6 Breaking up with a close friend.

At such times remember that your child needs a lot of understanding and support. Most of the, often distressing, changes in his or her behaviour which may occur are the result of attempting to cope with chronic stress.

In most cases things do resolve themselves, time heals painful wounds and your child adjusts to new circumstances. But if such an adjustment fails to occur the outcome could be burn-out.

BOSS – burn-out stress syndrome

The symptoms of BOSS to watch for in your child include;

- Exhaustion – loss of energy and rapid fatigue. There is a loss of trust, interest and concern for others.
- A decline in personal relationships and negative responses to other people. Your child is increasingly irritable, incapable of handling minor frustrations and much more inclined to focus on any failures than successes.
- Depression, frequent crying, poor self-esteem and feelings of hopelessness.
- Health problems, including upset digestion, aching muscles (especially in the lower back and neck), headaches and missed menstrual periods.

Once established, BOSS becomes a self-reinforcing process, as the negative attitudes and actions which result lead to further discouragement and withdrawal.

Mike's story

Mike, a pale, rather serious-looking twelve-year-old was brought to see me because he was showing many of the symptoms described above. Like Martin, whose difficulties I recounted in Chapter One, he was constantly tired, his appetite was poor and he slept badly.

It turned out that Mike's main anxiety focused on the bullying of a particular teacher, a burly, ex-army sergeant named Bob, who taught carpentry, metalwork and football. He made no secret of despising small, weedy, non-athletic boys, and from the very first lesson set out to make Mike's life a misery. He constantly picked on, belittled and humiliated him in front of the others. During games he mocked and ridiculed him constantly, often following him into the changing-room and causing laughter among the other boys by his sarcastic comments on Mike's scrawny frame.

Before long Mike came to dread his classes to such an extent that he began having nightmares about them. The stress created by this anxiety undermined his health so much that he constantly felt unwell. This only made him more vulnerable to other stresses. At about this time his parents' marriage went through a bad patch and they frequently rowed. His father often came home late and slightly drunk. In this condition he was extremely critical of Mike, going through his homework and making disparaging comments.

The boy became deeply depressed and chronically anxious. His academic work, at which he had previously excelled, suffered badly and he was moved out of the top stream into a class of much less able students. This left him humiliated and bored. Had nothing been done to help him, his whole future could have been placed in jeopardy by the activities of that one, sadistic, master.

Anxiety is not an illness

Before concluding this chapter, let me emphasise one crucial point. Anxiety is not an illness.

June's first thought when she suddenly found herself unable to pour out a cup of coffee was that she must have a serious physical complaint. Mike's parents concluded that their son must be mentally ill. They found it hard to believe that any child could behave as curiously as he did without there being some medical problem. Max, the fifteen-year-old whose examination nerves I described in Chapter One, was petrified by his anxieties. Extremely religious parents had convinced him that masturbating was a terrible sin, and he saw the panic attacks as God's punishment on him.

Sally, the spider phobic, believed that her fears were due to a weakness of character and lack of 'moral fibre' – a phrase her father had used in an attempt to 'shame' her out of her phobia. Since she was incapable of not feeling terror at the sight of a spider, this only made her feel even more inadequate.

It is not unreasonable for anxious people, especially children, to try and explain their humiliating and seemingly inexplicable fears in a wide variety of ways. But, hardly surprisingly, explanations based on the idea of having a serious physical illness (June), being mentally ill (Mike), the victim of God's wrath (Max) or a spineless ninny (Sally) only make the anxiety worse.

Some children, and adults, are more generally anxious than others. Because of the way their nervous systems are structured they respond more readily to anything which seems stressful. But this does not mean that they are weak or sick. As I explained in the last chapter, it could merely be a result of the way in which their genetic blueprint has put them together.

Anxiety, whether acute or chronic, is a natural response which is occurring either inappropriately – because what triggers it does not pose any genuine threat to your child's survival, as in the case of Sally's fear of spiders – or because it is appropriate but excessive. Virtually all children have some exam nerves, but Max's anxiety was out of all proportion to the situation.

The plan outlined in this book allows you to tackle both types of anxiety with equal success. The starting point, in every case, is to discover just what is going wrong. How that can be done I shall explain in the next chapter.

Four
Your Child's Hidden Fears

You know something is going wrong in your child's life because she has suddenly changed from being confident and outgoing to being difficult, insecure and withdrawn. Classroom achievement and an eagerness to learn have been replaced by failure and a dislike of school.

She has become a loner, shunning her old friends yet unwilling to make new ones. She has become moody, irritable or depressed. Yet nothing seems to have happened that would explain these changes, and your every attempt to discover what's causing that unhappiness is met with denial or even hostility. Your child either insists that *nothing* is wrong or tries to fob you off with an unsatisfactory answer.

As we shall see in a moment, these common responses to adult queries are one of the ways in which children protect themselves from becoming even more anxious.

To illustrate the type of exchanges which so often occur when parents attempt to probe the reasons behind their child's anxieties, let's eavesdrop on a conversation between thirteen-year-old Samantha and her mother, Jean. Over the past few weeks, Samantha, usually a cheerful, outgoing child, has grown increasingly moody and withdrawn. Several times recently Jean has discovered her sobbing her eyes out in her bedroom.

She no longer goes out to play with friends, and spends a lot of time alone. Now Jean has decided that it's high time for a heart-to-heart talk so she can get to the bottom of her daughter's obvious unhappiness. Sharing the washing-up after Sunday lunch gives Jean her opportunity.

She asks gently: 'What is it, Sam, why are you so miserable these days?'

Samantha frowns, shrugs her shoulders and says casually: 'Nothing's wrong. Everything's OK.'

Despite this discouraging response, and an expression on her daughter's face which warns her to change the subject, Jean persists: 'But you've been so miserable and moody lately. Is something wrong at school? Are you worried about your work?'

'No,' snaps Samantha.

'Have you had a row with one of your friends? Is that it?'

Samantha simply frowns and shrugs impatiently.

Jean says: 'This can't go on, can it?'

'What can't go on?'

'Your moods, staying in your room for hours on end, never seeing your friends, crying all the time.'

'I do not. When do I cry?'

'You know you've been crying. Please tell me what's wrong, so I can help.'

'There's nothing wrong,' Sam says loudly. 'I keep telling you, why don't you listen . . .'

'Look, I'm not trying to pry,' Jean tries to reassure her, 'but you must admit you've been acting strangely just recently. I'm worried . . .'

'Well, I'm sorry if I'm a burden to you,' Samantha yells.

Mother and daughter face each other like combatants and Jean is close to losing her temper. She makes one more attempt to get at the truth. Keeping her voice calm with difficulty she tells her daughter: 'I love you darling. I only want you to be happy. That's why I'm so concerned . . .'

'You're always picking on me, getting at me. Just leave me alone can't you . . . leave me alone . . .' Samantha shouts, and Jean's anger gets the better of her.

'How dare you speak to me like that. Go to your room at once.'

With a sob, Samantha flings down the drying-up cloth and runs from the kitchen. Jean hears the bedroom door slam, and the child's muffled tears as she flings herself on to the bed in despair.

Sound familiar?

That exchange was typical of scores I have recorded while working with parents and children. Later in this chapter we'll look at what was going on in more detail by identifying the type of defence mechanisms which an already highly anxious Samantha was using to protect herself from further anxiety. In the next chapter I'll be explaining the right way to hold that kind of a conversation, but, for the moment, let's explore some of the reasons why a child may try to keep anxieties and fears hidden from view.

Why children hide their anxieties

As adults we know how helpful it can be to talk with close friends or relatives, to unburden ourselves to a doctor, psychologist or priest. Just voicing anxieties somehow makes them less frightening and more manageable. We firmly believe in that old saying about a burden shared being a burden halved. So why should children frequently want to keep their worries hidden from loving parents?

The best way of answering this common query is to ask another question in return. Would you be willing to reveal your anxieties to a friend or relative if the person in whom you confided:

- was in a position to punish you for speaking out?
- couldn't be trusted not to spread your confessions all over the neighbourhood?
- might be so worried by what you said that her own health and happiness suffered?
- would not understand or have any sympathy for your anxieties?
- was liable to use your admissions against you at a later date?
- could feel so upset that he, or she, would never want to see you again?
- might regard you as disgusting or perverted?
- was likely to make matters worse by well-meaning but incompetent attempts to help?

The answer is, of course, 'No'. In fact you'd almost certainly go to great lengths to keep your anxieties secret. And if the other person kept demanding that you discuss those problems, you'd probably feel angry and resentful. You'd tell them to mind their own business and start avoiding them.

Many children feel the same way about their parents. On past experience of confessing secret thoughts and deeds they fear punishment, rejection, humiliation, criticism, sarcasm, a lack of understanding, a tendency to make their difficulties worse through ill-advised meddling. In short, they stay silent from fear. On top of their original anxiety they are also anxious about having to discuss what is making them fearful.

Anxieties that keep your child silent

Here are some of the major anxieties children have about admitting their anxieties to grown-ups:

- Not being taken seriously.
- Appearing silly, babyish, incompetent or unmanly.
- Being teased, ridiculed or humiliated. After Sally, the nine-year-old spider phobic I discussed in Chapter One, admitted her fear of spiders, she was mocked by her parents in what they fondly believed was their daughter's own best interest. They hoped that she could be 'shamed' out of her phobia. When her fellow pupils found out they teased her, and ended up playing a cruel practical joke.
- Embarrassment, guilt or shame. This is especially likely when anxieties are due to anything which is a taboo topic in the family, such as nudity or sex.

  Fifteen-year-old Max, whose exam fears led to school failure, was petrified by his 'wet dreams', convinced that the nocturnal emissions were a symptom of some venereal disease. Yet he dared not reveal these worries to his extremely religious parents out of a greater fear that they would consider him degenerate.

  In more extreme cases, youngsters who are being sexually abused may remain silent throughout years of torment, both through a terror of what the abusing grown-up might do to

them, shame over what they are being compelled to do and fear that nobody will believe them if they do try and explain.
- Making things worse. For example, where bullying, by an older child or a teacher, is involved, the child may worry that attempts to help will get him branded as a 'sneak' or 'Mummy's boy'. Children involved in gang activities are often terrified of reprisals if they tell you what has happened. Children being abused or assaulted by grown-ups keep their grim secret, often for years and sometimes all their lives, for this reason too.
- Concern that the secret will get around and his friends will mock or think badly of him.
- Anxiety that the confession will be used against him during future rows or disagreements. This is by no means a rare occurrence, especially during bitter family rows. I overheard one mother tell her 10-year-old son: 'You think you're grown . . . what kind of big man is still scared of the dark?'

Why children have such anxieties

You may feel that no loving parent would do any of the things I've described; that, however dreadful the truth, they would surely go on supporting and caring for their child.

Sadly, that is by no means always true. Parents can and do reject their children, or at least give a very good impression of doing so, if their conduct outrages the parents' most deeply held beliefs.

Phillipa, a fifteen-year-old, became involved with a gang of girls who went shoplifting in their lunch hour. A previously honest girl with deeply religious parents, she stopped after a couple of stealing expeditions, disgusted with herself for being so dishonest. Her distress at having gone against all she believed in made Phillipa so anxious that she became physically ill.

Her parents implored her to tell them what was wrong, and insisted that they would still love and stand by her no matter how dreadful the truth. But when she did, finally, confess to stealing, her father – whom she loved very deeply – strode from the room without a word. From that day to the time she was seventeen and left home, he refused to speak to her again.

Although such extreme reactions are rare, the important point is what a child believes *could* happen as a result of explaining the reasons for his anxiety. Even if there is only a tiny chance of any of those unpleasant consequences occurring, most children prefer to stay silent than take the risk. Confessing is like pulling the trigger of a loaded gun. The spoken word can no more be recalled than a speeding bullet.

To make matters worse, excessively anxious children have poor judgement. Their anxiety makes them overly timid, with a poor self-image, little confidence and a great reluctance to take any kind of risk. They feel so vulnerable to criticism or rejection that they go to great lengths to avoid it. Their anxiety also makes them particularly sensitive to anything connected with their fears. Sally, the spider phobic, for instance, would instantly notice even the tiniest spider in an otherwise spotless room. Twelve-year-old Mike's dread of bullying made him immediately aware of the slightest increase in tension within a group of children. The merest suggestion of disagreement, irritation or aggression was enough to make him extremely apprehensive.

One final barrier to disclosure is an inability to put anxieties into words. Even when they want to explain what's going wrong in their lives, many younger children are unable to put their fears into words because they lack the language skills needed to express deeply felt emotions.

Anxiety can be disguised

So far we've assumed that you recognise your child to be suffering from an anxiety problem. But it may also be that a child is extremely anxious for a long period without your realising the fact. This is because the way in which children choose to defend themselves against their anxieties can cause these to emerge in disguised forms which seem to have nothing to do with anxiety.

Let's look at the seven most common disguises which anxiety can assume. While reading the list, reflect on how many you would have attributed to anxiety, and how many to your child being lazy, naughty, impulsive, unintelligent, impudent or rebellious?

1: Avoidance

One of the most commonly used defences against anxiety is avoiding the things which make us anxious. Your child has a monthly maths test which, as he is bad at the subject, causes great anxiety. Each month, on test day, he gets a headache, stomach pains, a snuffly nose or sore throat. Sometimes you are sufficiently concerned to keep him at home, when his anxiety instantly vanishes and unpleasant feelings are replaced by a sense of relief.

In this way the avoidance is rewarded, making it more likely that he'll adopt the same strategy the next time around. And, of course, by missing those tests he falls even further behind, gets still more confused and so find that the tests provoke even greater anxiety. It is through this pattern of avoidance and reward that a phobia often develops.

In extreme cases, avoidance can lead to truancy or school refusal, either on a regular basis or only during those days when some particularly anxiety-arousing activity is on the timetable.

Where physical avoidance is impossible, your child may resort to intellectual or emotional avoidance. There are two ways of doing this. The first is to escape into a pleasant world of daydreams whenever an anxiety-arousing subject is being discussed. The child who is fearful of geography, for instance, may intellectually absent herself from the lesson as soon as the teacher starts speaking. By doing so, of course, she misses the key points, falls further behind the rest of the class and is thus made even more anxious on subsequent lessons.

When children tell you 'I can't do . . .', and then list all the subjects they find incomprehensible, it's a fair bet that anxiety is involved. They are avoiding the need even to attempt any understanding of the subject by closing their minds to it.

By comparison, children who say, 'I don't know how to . . .', and then list the subjects they find hard, are not made anxious by their lack of ability. On the contrary, they are confident that understanding will come in time.

For 'can't doers' the world is filled with impossibilities; for 'don't knowers' it is full of possibilities.

The single most important step which any parent or teacher ever takes is to transform an underachieving child from the attitude of mind which says 'can't know' to one of 'don't know'. But until the anxiety responsible for that escape into the comfortable world of 'can't know' has been removed, the essential change of outlook can never occur.

Emotional avoidance is achieved by a refusal to face up to those anxiety-arousing feelings. This is a special problem for boys raised in homes where it is considered unmanly to show your emotions and, especially, to weep. Such children not only suffer the anxiety created by a sad event, but also further anxiety caused by a conflict between the way they want to respond, with grief and tears, and the way they are expected to react, by putting on a 'brave face' and showing a 'stiff upper lip'. In a short time this avoidance leads to what psychologists have, rather inelegantly, called 'emotional constipation'.

Its effect is a blocking-up of feelings, as though their emotional mechanisms had been anaesthetised. Not only does this make it very hard for them to relate to other people, especially those who have no inhibitions over revealing their emotions, but the tensions get bottled up inside. At some point the pressure becomes so great that it causes an explosion, often with disastrous consequences.

As I have previously mentioned, impulsive children are often anxious children. They use the speed of their response as an avoidance strategy. Given a difficult problem to solve, for instance, they will race through it without allowing their brain any time to ponder the questions.

In one study, a group of thirteen- and fourteen-year-olds from the bottom stream of a secondary school were asked to attempt a demanding IQ test. Known as the AH4 after its creator, psychologist Alice Heim, this is normally given to university students, who find it a considerable intellectual challenge.

Yet these underachieving teenagers raced through the

problems, finishing far earlier than undergraduates and being much more confident of their level of attainment. In fact they had failed to answer more questions correctly than predicted by chance alone. In other words their number of right answers would have been significantly higher had they shut their eyes and stuck a pin into the question paper! Their anxiety had been so great that they avoided applying anything but the most rapid thought to the test.

Aggression, too, can often be traced to anxiety avoidance. A child who has been teased by another may be made so anxious that he lashes out in an attempt to end the torment. In school, a child made anxious by his inability to understand lessons may start acting the clown. This provides a distraction from the painful task of trying to comprehend the seemingly incomprehensible, gives him attention otherwise denied, and could even result in his being expelled from the room – so providing the relief of physical avoidance.

Be on the look out for anxiety which comes in the guise of:

• Avoidance, whether physical or mental – a refusal to attempt anxiety-arousing activities or express certain feelings.
• Impulsiveness – a desire to get the feared task or confrontation over as quickly as possible.
• Aggression – a way of bringing anxiety to an end by physical means.

2: *Projection*
This is the name given to the very human failing of blaming others for our own mistakes. For instance, the incompetent boss who always places responsibility for blunders on to his 'stupid' subordinates, or the teacher who shifts the blame for poor examination results on to her 'lazy, dull' students.

By projecting our own inadequacies on to others, the anxiety which mistakes and misjudgements arouse can be reduced. Children made anxious by school failure may blame their lack of success on poor teaching, crowded classrooms, insufficient support from parents and so on. While there is often some truth in such allegations, children who are achieving well under identical circumstances seldom regard any of them as being much of a problem.

If your child starts sounding off about how useless her school is, how bad the teachers are and how difficult it is to work in noisy classrooms, you could certainly investigate her complaints. But at the same time bear in mind that at least part of the problem may lie in her own attitudes, and that these attitudes could be strongly influenced by anxiety.

3: Repression

Here anxiety-arousing ideas, feelings, thoughts or experiences are hidden away deep in the unconscious. Although no longer accessible, without special help, to conscious thought, they continue to exert a profound influence over many aspects of one's life. Freud believed that adult neuroses stem from early, fearful, memories which have been repressed because they are too distressing to think about.

I remember one attractive young woman who came to see me reporting an intense fear of sex. Although she liked men and enjoyed their company, as soon as the relationship seemed to be getting serious she would immediately stop seeing the man.

In her case the repressed fear, which emerged during therapy, was of a man exposing himself to her when she was playing in a wood near her home at the age of four. She had never told anybody of this incident, which remained repressed for more than sixteen years. Yet, below the surface of her mind, the anxiety it created was powerful enough to make her terrified of ever seeing another naked man.

4: Displacement

Here, anxiety over one thing is shifted or displaced on to something else. Your child is struggling with homework and getting more and more wound up. Suddenly she explodes in fury and the books go flying across the room. In this way the tensions and anxieties created by not being able to understand her work are released via an act of destruction. The same defence mechanism is at work when a child who is anxious about making friends resorts to bullying or telling fantastic stories in order to make other children pay attention to him.

5: *Rationalisation*

This is the 'sour grapes' strategy for defending oneself against anxiety. You may remember the famous Aesop fable in which the fox, being unable to eat some grapes, comforted himself with the thought that they were in any case probably too sour to enjoy.

Your child can't have something, so he decides that it wasn't worth having in the first place. Many of the negative attitudes found among older school children stem from this mechanism. It works like this: the child feels incapable of getting good exam grades and knows he is going to be branded a failure. This makes him very anxious. To defend himself, he decides that exams aren't worth passing, school is a waste of time, adults know nothing about the real world and so on.

6: *Undoing*

This is a term used by Freud to describe those little pieces of ritual magic which virtually everybody uses to defend themselves against the anxiety created by uncertainty. Your child is attending an important interview, so she insists on wearing her 'lucky' dress or carrying a good-luck charm. Or perhaps he tells himself that he'll pass the chemistry exam if all the traffic lights on the drive to school are green.

Undoing does no harm in moderation, but it can have two unfortunate consequences for a child who uses this as a regular means of managing anxiety.

Firstly, it creates a belief that destiny is all a matter of chance, fate and luck. That he can do little, except by placating the goddess of fortune with little rituals, to control what happens to him, what success he enjoys, what goals he accomplishes. Not only does this lead to a sense of helplessness – itself a source of considerable anxiety – but it may also prevent a child from taking the practical steps needed to bring about desired changes in an unhappy or unsatisfactory situation.

A child who fails an exam, for instance, may convince herself that it was because she forgot her 'lucky' pencil or couldn't sit at her 'lucky' seat in the examination room. Instead of looking at what needs to be improved in her study, revision or exam taking skills, she dismisses the outcome as the result of 'bad luck'.

A second problem is that these rituals may eventually start dominating your child's life. This could produce compulsive behaviour that makes it almost impossible to live normally. He may spend hours each day washing his hands, for instance, or be unable to sleep unless every picture and poster in his bedroom is hanging dead straight.

7: Denial

When given bad news our immediate reaction is often to gasp, 'Oh, no . . . it's not true.' Sometimes, after her spouse has died, an elderly woman will continue to set him a place at table, or convince herself that he is going to come home as usual that evening.

A child uses denial of reality for the same reasons – to protect himself or herself against anxiety. Children whose school record is so poor that they will have great difficulty in finding work may deny that exam grades matter. Similarly, a child whose parents are on the point of separating might insist that they are a happy, united family.

Parents use the same strategy to deal with anxiety aroused by their children's behaviour. The mother of a glue-sniffer, for instance, refused to accept the reality of her child's addiction even when presented with clear evidence.

If your child is clearly miserable, yet refuses to acknowledge that he is upset or unhappy, denial may be responsible. Having to tell you about his fears would mean bringing them out into the open where their reality could no longer be hidden from him. By saying: 'No, honestly . . . there's nothing wrong. I'm OK, really I am . . .' he prevents himself from being overwhelmed by his anxieties.

If you insist that something *is* making him anxious and demand to know what it is, he may resort to some of the other strategies we've looked at.

Running from the room reduces anxiety through physical avoidance. Provoking a fight with you, as Samantha did, by yelling: 'You're always picking on me, getting at me. Just leave me alone, can't you . . . leave me alone . . .' usually lets your child off the hook. It may make you feel so anxious, or guilty, that you rapidly change the subject. Or it could bring the conversation to an end by causing you, as it did Samantha's mother Jean, to lose your temper and yell: 'How dare you speak to me like that. Go to your room at once.' As with Samantha, your child exits, miserable but with his denial mechanism still intact.

Blaming his problems on you, or your partner, or somebody else allows the denial to persist. 'It's all your fault . . . you've never understood me,' she yells. Because most parents seem burdened down by more than their fair share of guilt, that accusation often hits home and diverts the adult from pursuing the cause of the anxiety any further.

As you can see, anxiety can find many forms of expression, many of which are rarely recognised as having anything to do with feeling anxious.

Defences can be positive

Although harmful when they get in the way of identifying and dealing with anxiety problems, defence mechanisms have a positive value under the right circumstances.

Take avoidance, for example. Unhelpful when it stops a child from confronting and conquering an anxiety-arousing challenge, it is also an essential survival mechanism. Your child must learn to avoid genuinely dangerous situations – like the stranger who offers a lift home or the bully who might cause serious injury.

Similarly, rationalisation allows children to analyse their experiences, anticipate outcomes and seek alternative ways of behaving.

Displacement enables them to change or modify their behaviour in the light of changed situations. A child who gets wound up in a row, for instance, can release that tension in a positive and acceptable way by displacing it into a sports activity. A child made anxious by his teacher's criticisms may displace his feelings into a determination to work harder and show the critic what a mistake she made.

Repression of many anti-social impulses is an essential qualification for living in a civilised society. The child who has no control over his or her emotions will obviously find it very hard to get on in life.

Denial is a means of selectively focusing one's attention so that important issues can be attended to without harmful distraction. It is usually more helpful to adults than children. For example, a doctor working with seriously ill patients must 'deny' much of the pain suffered by victims if she is to keep her head and do her job professionally.

What makes your child anxious?

Now that we've considered the different forms anxiety can take, let's look at the six major causes of such anxiety, together with the defence mechanisms most often used to cope with them.

Meeting grown-ups' expectations

This is most likely if you, or your child's teachers, are over perfectionist or give the impression, however unintentionally, that love or respect for the child depends on sustained achievement.

However, such anxieties also occur even when no apparent pressure is put on the child to succeed. Here the drive toward success comes from within, sometimes as a result of the child striving to match the attainments of an older brother or sister, or simply because he or she is being raised in a family where achievement is taken for granted.

What matters is how your child perceives the importance of success and the ways in which failures are dealt with. As I shall explain in a later chapter, children can strive for success either from a need for achievement or out of a fear of failure. The former is a positive force which allows children to learn from their setbacks and not be made over anxious by their mistakes. But where a child is motivated by a desire to avoid failing at any cost, the emotional cost of each success is high and the price paid for errors and blunders excessive.

Defence mechanisms commonly used. Avoidance. Projection. Displacement. Rationalisation. Undoing. Denial.

Family feelings
Some children are made very anxious by even trivial rows between their parents. If your marriage is going through a difficult patch, a mutual agreement never to fight in front of the children does nothing to remove those fears.

Children are skilled at reading body language, and know intuitively when the emotional atmosphere is tense and angry. Indeed, when parents deny that anything is wrong, and the child's instinct tells him that all is far from well, the resulting anxiety can be even worse. Matters are often made worse because adult motives and actions can easily be misunderstood or misinterpreted. A minor squabble with your partner, which you quickly forget, may be seen as very serious by an already anxious child. Truancy is often a result of fears about what may happen at home while the child is away, rather than anxiety over what is going on in school.

Remember that once a child has developed an anxiety he or she will be particularly sensitive to anything which tends to lend support to that worry, while less attentive to evidence which contradicts it. If the child believes that Mum and Dad are on bad terms, every frown, sigh and irritable retort will be noticed, while signs of affection, tenderness or empathy may be overlooked.

Defence mechanisms commonly used. Avoidance. Projection. Repression, Rationalisation. Denial.

Sexual anxieties
While these are, occasionally, caused by an actual assault, they are more usually provoked by explicit sex scenes on TV or on surreptitiously viewed X-rated videos, sexual horseplay between older children, smutty jokes or the boasts of more mature companions.

They can also be caused by a conflict between activities which the child finds pleasurable and parental condemnation. Even very small children experience much enjoyment from touching and rubbing their genitals, and have great sexual curiosity. Playing 'doctors and nurses', or exhibiting their body to children of the same or opposite sex, seems perfectly natural to them. The often excessive adult response to such activities, however, creates guilt, fear and anxiety.

Defence mechanisms commonly used. Avoidance. Repression. Displacement. Rationalisation. Denial.

Bullying
If there are no obvious signs of physical violence, such as a bleeding nose or black eye, it can be hard to accept that bullying is a problem. But even threats of aggression from a stronger child may terrify a less assertive youngster. Sarcasm, teasing and being made the class scapegoat can cause both boys and girls considerable anxiety.

Defence mechanisms commonly used. Avoidance. Projection. Displacement. Denial.

Their own health
Young children may develop this anxiety as a result of not properly understanding health instruction in class or as a result of scare stories in the newspapers and on TV. Like first-year medical students, they assume every ache and pain is the symptom of a serious illness. Adult remarks which were intended as a joke, such as 'if you eat any more your stomach will burst' may be taken seriously by a child already anxious about his health.

Defence mechanisms commonly used. Projection. Denial. Repression.

Violence and nuclear war
Studies have shown that one in three children worry about nuclear war, terrorists, burglars and muggers. Children are especially vulnerable to such anxieties between the ages of around six and ten, because, although old enough to be aware of life's dangers, they lack the judgement and maturity to put their fears into perspective.

Violence and suffering are viewed nightly on television, unpleasant things happen in school, they know that grown-ups fight and families break up, yet they don't have the understanding needed to handle the anxiety this knowledge arouses. The answer is not to censor their viewing, although discretion should always be exercised about exposing young children to violent or disturbing material, but to assist them in evaluating the level of personal risk more accurately.

Defence mechanisms commonly used. Avoidance. Denial. Rationalisation. Repression.

Putting it all together

In this chapter we have seen that anxiety may be carefully concealed, even from sympathetic and caring adults, for a variety of reasons which seem important to the child. This can make it hard to discover the cause of your child's anxieties and fears.

Furthermore, the use of various defence mechanisms may cause anxiety to emerge in a disguised form. Seven of these were described in Chapter Four. Among the many guises anxiety can assume are moodiness, irritability, aggressive behaviour, sulking, classroom failure, obstinacy, rebellion, truancy, temper tantrums, sarcasm and various forms of 'naughtiness'.

Under these circumstances adults are more likely to attribute such feelings and actions to causes like disobedience, depravity, impulsiveness, immaturity, insolence, laziness, rebellion, rudeness, selfishness, stupidity and wickedness.

Recognising that anxiety *could* be the reason for your child's changed outlook, attitude or behaviour is the first stage in helping to free him or her from these distressing feelings. The second stage is to pinpoint the likely cause, or causes, of that anxiety. I shall explain how this can be done in Chapter Five.

Part Two
Exploring your child's anxieties

Five
Discovering Your Child's Anxieties

In this chapter I shall tell you how to take the first of three steps towards helping your child banish distressing and disabling anxieties. To accomplish this you must find answers to three vital questions: 'Is my child suffering from excessive anxiety?' If the answer is yes, the next question is: 'which area of his or her life is creating that anxiety?' Having established the general area, for instance school, leisure activities or home life, you must try to pinpoint the source of the difficulties more precisely by discovering: 'Which specific activities or situations arouse the greatest anxiety?'

I'll start by explaining how you can discover whether anxiety could be at the root of your child's problems or failures.

Step One: Is anxiety the problem?

Sometimes this is an easy question to answer. Sally's parents, for instance, knew from the start that their daughter was terrified of spiders. But frequently, for the reasons outlined in the last chapter, it is less clear whether a child's difficulties are a result of anxiety or fear.

As we have seen, the ways in which people defend themselves from anxiety mean that it can appear in several guises: moodiness, irritability, aggressive behaviour, impulsiveness, sulking, disruptive conduct, obstinacy, rebellion, truancy and temper tantrums.

In such cases parents and teachers are more inclined to lay the blame on laziness, lack of intelligence, disobedience and other kinds of 'naughtiness' than on anxiety.

Step Two: Which area of life is creating the anxiety?

Again, this question is not always as easy to answer as it sounds. Even when you know *how* anxiety is affecting your child's behaviour, for instance by spoiling her chances of success during examinations, it does not necessarily mean that you have identified the cause of the trouble. Here's an example of how one can easily be deceived.

After moving to a higher stream in maths, twelve-year-old Alison started falling badly behind. She was clearly being made very anxious by the challenge of a much tougher course. Her father, convinced that her anxiety was due to a lack of understanding, arranged for his daughter to have extra coaching. Instead of improving she actually started doing worse. Even more puzzling was her tutor's report that Alison understood the subject very well and answered almost every test question correctly when not under any pressure to do so.

The true causes of the maths anxieties were later found to lie not the classroom at all, but at home. They arose from Alison's relationship with a demanding and over-perfectionist father. His critical attitude and high expectations so terrified the girl that, whenever she felt herself being put to the test, anxiety soared and performance nose-dived.

I also remember a woman client in her twenties who, after a brilliant start to her school career, had fallen behind academically and finally left without any worthwhile qualifications. She recalled vividly the moment at which she gave up trying to please her parents by doing well in school. She had worked extremely hard at chemistry, a subject she disliked, and had come third out of a class of sixty students. Her mother's only response to this achievement was a sneering comment that they weren't interested in the third-raters and the only place worth having was first. 'After that I just stopped working at all,' she told me. 'It didn't seem worth the effort.'

In other cases children have deliberately failed because they were made so anxious about appearing brighter than their less achieving friends, or being ridiculed as a 'teacher's pet'. One very gifted fourteen-year-old boy was always coming home with bruises, cuts and the occasional black eye. His mother told me that she knew he always mixed with the roughest, meanest and least academically achieving group of boys in the school.

'Why don't you make friends with clever boys like yourself,' she once asked him, 'rather than those toughs?'

'It's hard enough to survive there if you've got brains,' he replied. 'My only hope is to stay friendly with the toughs.'

A less confident child might have simply abandoned any attempt to be more intelligent than his companions.

Step Three: Which activities or situations within that life area arouse the greatest anxiety?

Once you have identified the general area in which anxieties are undermining happiness or success, the third and final stage is to pinpoint the specific people, situations or activities most likely to produce these negative feelings.

Suppose you discovered that your child's inability to make friends is due to anxiety about dealing with any new or novel situation. Since each meeting with strangers is just such a situation, your child has got into the habit of using avoidance ('I'm not going to that party!') and rationalisation ('Who needs friends anyhow?') as defences against the anxiety aroused. Until you have defined the problem more carefully, however, and focused on exactly those aspects of the situation which cause the greatest problems, you cannot be of much help.

What makes such challenges more or less anxiety-arousing? Does he find it easier to meet unfamiliar people in familiar settings than in strange surroundings? If the answer is 'yes', then he'll be more willing to hold a party at home than accept an invitation to one in somebody else's house.

Is there less anxiety when just one or two strangers are present or does she feel more relaxed when able to lose herself in a crowd? When creating a programme to help her overcome these fears, the answers to these questions could mean the difference between success and failure.

In order to answer these three questions you need to adopt different forms of assessment, though there is usually a certain overlap between them. When discovering that anxiety is the underlying problem, you sometimes also learn what areas of life are responsible. Similarly, identifying the general area of life involved generally provides clues as to the specific situations that arouse most anxiety.

In Step One, careful observation, combined with an analysis of your child's drawings, are the most useful strategies. For Step Two (detailed in Chapter Six), paper and pencil assessments can be helpful with older children. In the final Step (details in Chapter Seven), you will need to master the skill of positive listening.

Step One: Identifying anxiety as the problem

I have already described several ways in which your child may behave when suffering from either chronic or acute anxiety. The quiz in Chapter Two and my comments in Chapter Four should also be of help.

When it comes to systematic exploration of your child's anxieties, however, a written record of his or her behaviour, in the form of a special kind of diary, can prove extremely helpful.

Keeping a diary

There's no need to make long, detailed entries. Just note down what your child did that day, together with any signs of anxiety, such as loss of appetite, disturbed sleep, irritability, tears, tummy upsets and so on. Use the quiz in Chapter Two as a guide to the common bodily effects of anxiety.

The approach I recommend is called the ABC method, with each letter standing for the features to watch out for.

A = Antecedent. This means the events that happened immediately before your child showed signs of distress, anger, obstinacy, tearfulness and so on. Was some comment made or criticism offered? Did you ask, or tell, him to do something? Was it the day before she was due to take a test, play games, go swimming? Make a note of who else was present (i.e. brothers, sisters, friends, other relatives, etc.) time of day and where the incident happened.

You could find, for instance, that your child is more anxious when your partner or another child is present. He may be able to control his anxiety in the morning, when fresh from a night's rest, but prove far more vulnerable by evening, when he feels tired and drained. You could discover that certain rooms, or places, trigger anxieties. For example, after a car accident in which his sister was badly hurt, eleven-year-old Jason felt especially on edge when being driven to school. But because he was also anxious during breakfast, while anticipating the terrifying drive through town, and for a while after arriving at school, as he gradually wound down after the anxiety of the trip, it was not at all obvious what was causing his difficulty. The diary kept by his mother for ten days, together with the questions she was able to ask him based on that record, finally identified the true cause of his fears.

B = Behaviour. Note, as carefully as possible, what your child actually did. She might, for instance, have burst into tears and run out of the room. He may have yelled in fury and flung his homework across the room. Did he become more aggressive, hitting out or yelling his anger? Did she freeze up, becoming very quiet and almost motionless, avoiding anyone else's gaze or refusing to answer their questions?

C = Consequence. What happened as a result of that behaviour. Did it change the situation in some way that reduced your child's anxiety?

Here's how it might work. You tell your daughter about a party invitation (Antecedent). She makes a scene and refuses to go (Behaviour). You give in rather than risk a scene and tell her you'll phone with an excuse (Consequence).

After a week or ten days, read through the entries to see

whether your child's mood has been especially negative on certain days. Do days when there is a particular subject on the timetable cause special distress? Is homework specially stressful – and if so are all subjects equally bad, or does one cause far more heartache than the others?

Continue with the diary as you work with your child on the practical anxiety management plan described in the next chapter. This will enable you to monitor progress as the training progresses.

There is another very helpful, although usually neglected, source of information about your child's feelings and fears. These are the drawings and paintings he or she makes. By looking at the way illustrations are created, the themes chosen, and the colours used you can gain valuable insights into your child's outlook on life.

Art and your child's anxiety

To make this assessment you will need six drawings or paintings which your child has completed over the past few weeks that depict a human figure. If no such pictures are available ask for some to be drawn especially, but without saying how you intend to use them. These drawings should be produced over a period of days to prevent your child from getting bored and rushing the pictures.

They must be full-length portraits of six different people (age and sex are unimportant), drawn as carefully as your child is capable.

Examine the drawings for these six key features of anxiety;

1 Omissions
2 Distortions
3 Heavy pressure
4 Mouths turned down
5 Hands raised
6 Arms turned inward

Studies by Dr Leonard Handler of the University of Tennessee, and Dr Joseph Reyger of Michigan State University, have shown that these early identifiable features are associated with higher than average anxiety in children aged from five to fourteen.

Add up the number of features present in the drawings. The more there are the greater your child's underlying anxiety is likely to prove.

Omissions. These can be easy to spot, for instance missing hands or feet. At other times they are subtle and harder to detect, such as the absence of lips, eyebrows, fingers or ears, buttons left off a coat or laces from shoes.

The picture below was drawn by six-year-old Tania, who underwent a marked mood change after spending a few days in hospital for a minor operation. A once cheerful and enthusiastic child, she came home withdrawn and miserable. At first her parents assumed that this was due to natural weakness following surgery, but when it still persisted three months later they sought advice.

Tania's drawings not only revealed chronic anxiety but, as often happens, suggested a reason for her anxiety. A notable feature of the girl's work was her fascination with medicine. Over half her paintings, and many of her drawings, depicted hospitals, doctors, nurses or patients. She painted ambulances racing up to the casualty department, wards filled with bandaged patients and white-coated doctors.

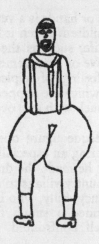

Whenever an anxious child seems obsessed by a particular theme it is likely that the subject matter reflects her anxieties. Tania's pictures suggested that her mood change could be caused by anxiety over the possibility of being sent back to hospital.

Using the technique of *positive listening*, which I shall describe in Chapter Seven, her parents were able to identify this as the reason for her unhappiness. Being too young properly to understand why she had been sent to hospital in the first place, Tania came to believe that it must be a punishment for being naughty. On returning home she was terrified that, if she was ever a bad girl again, her parents would send her back. Once convinced that her fears were groundless, Tania's anxiety disappeared and she was soon her old happy and self-assured self again.

Tania's pictures show three significant omissions. See if you can spot what they are before reading on – this is good practice for analysing your own child's pictures. Here they are:

1 Both arms are missing.
2 There is no mouth – but she's left a gap for it in the beard.
3 The eyes have no pupils.

The absence of arms or hands is a very common feature of pictures by anxious children. Often it links to some kind of crisis in that child's life, such as the break-up of a close friendship, a house move or bereavement. The lack of hands symbolises the child's feelings of helplessness, his inability to control the bad things which are happening to him. His sense of being both out of touch with and overwhelmed by life.

Distortions. The grotesque figure opposite was drawn by eight-year-old Billy, during an especially anxious time in his life. Six months before he made the drawings, Billy's family moved from a small country village to a large city as a result of his father's redundancy. Billy, who had lived all his life in the country and attended a small, friendly, local school suddenly found himself confronted with the anonymous

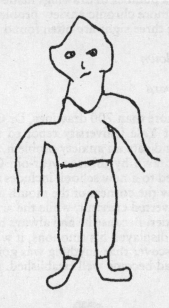

bustle of city life. Instead of being among friends in a small school, he found himself lonely and isolated in a huge and impersonal comprehensive.

Many of the drawings he made around this time contained distortions, as well as other indications of his acute anxiety.

Heavy pressure. To detect this sign of anxiety, run your fingers gently along the underside of the drawing. Provided the paper is of normal weight, you'll be able to detect any heavy pencil pressure by the ridges made in the paper. These are the result of muscle tensions leading to excess force being applied while forming the lines.

Such needless pressure is a clear indication that the child was under greater than normal stress when the drawing was made. You can't, of course, place much reliance on a single drawing since the stress might have been temporary, perhaps even caused by having to make the drawing in a hurry or while momentarily angry or anxious. But where pressure persists through a number of drawings made over a period of days or weeks a more chronic anxiety problem is suggested.

The remaining three signs are often found together.

Mouths turned down
Hands raised
Arms turned inward

After studying more than 700 drawings, Dr Cynthia Fox and her colleagues at Yale University reported that these three features clearly indicate an anxiety problem.

This picture, drawn by thirteen-year-old Colin soon after he had transferred to a new school, includes two of the three signs. Notice how the corners of the mouth are turned down to produce an inverted crescent, while the arms are raised as though in surrender. Because he had always been a rather shy boy, who rarely displayed his emotions, it was very hard for his parents to discover that anything was going wrong, until the difficulties had become well established.

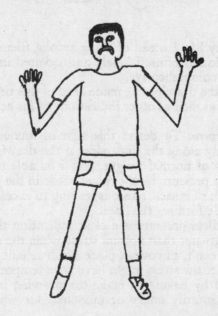

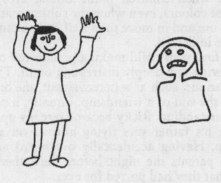

Colin had become the victim of a cruel 'protection racket' run by a gang of older boys. They demanded weekly payments in return for not roughing up the younger boys. Colin had been secretly stealing money from his parents to make these payments. Not only was he terrified of the gang, but he was also fearful about stealing from his parents. Colin's father had caught and punished him for taking money some weeks earlier. Even then he had been too afraid to explain what had caused his dishonesty, and continued to steal after being found out.

If your child's drawings include a turned-down mouth, arms raised more than 45 degrees above the body, or hands turned inwards – as illustrated above – high levels of anxiety are suggested.

Even when only one of these three features occurs regularly in your child's drawings you should take steps to find out if anything is making him or her particularly anxious or fearful.

Colour and anxiety. So far we have looked at drawings, but the colours used when painting can be equally helpful in identifying an anxiety problem. Of special significance is the use of purple or black as the dominant colour in a picture. By 'dominant colour', I mean one that is used extensively in the picture even when the subject matter does not demand it. A black night sky or purple robes on a king would be perfectly normal. But when children paint almost everything with either of these colours, even when the subject matter does not dictate their use and in more than half their pictures, anxiety problems are indicated.

You may find your child making greater use of black and purple following any deeply distressing event. This could be something serious, such as a bereavement, the break-up of a marriage or the end of a friendship. Equally, it could be due to a misunderstanding. Ricky became terribly upset when he learned that his father was flying abroad on an extended business trip. Having accidentally overheard an argument between his parents the night before his father left, Ricky concluded that they had parted for ever.

The seeds of this terrifying notion had been sown in his mind by the separation of his best friend's parents a few weeks earlier. His despair at the thought of never seeing his father again led to a spate of dismal, black-dominated paintings. Being shy and not very articulate, Ricky found it impossible to tell his mother about this worry. Only on seeing her son's paintings did she realise that something was wrong, manage to discover the cause of his unhappiness and offer him the reassurance he needed.

Where purple and black dominate your child's pictures for months the colours reveal not just a passing mood of anxiety but a generally unhappy, depressed and pessimistic outlook on life. Such children need support, reassurance and guidance to resolve the conflicts responsible for these painful emotions.

Red is the colour of aggression, and when it dominates more than half your child's paintings, especially if not required by the subject matter, there is good reason for supposing an above-average level of aggression. But remember that being aggressive is often a mask for anxiety, with the child seeking either to bring to an end something which makes him feel anxious, or preventing it from occurring in the first place. The boy who hits his sister because she has been mocking him, may well be using an aggressive response to stop his humiliation. The child who bullies other children at parties may be doing so because he has never learned a better way of coping with social anxieties.

Overpainting. Here, after completing the picture, a child paints over parts of it with another colour. For instance, a blue sky might be overpainted red, a green lawn smeared with yellow, or a red house daubed in black.

This means that the emotions expressed by the first colour are being concealed by feelings associated with the second. If, for instance, your child overpaints red with purple or black, it may indicate that anxiety and depression are being used to mask anger or hostility.

Where yellow, a colour linked to happy, joyous feelings, has been overpainted with green, indicating emotional restraint, your child may be attempting to hide positive emotions, perhaps for fear of having them destroyed by a careless word or deed.

Understanding the nature of overpainting will give you a helpful insight into your child's inhibitions and conflicts.

Why, for example, does the child who paints black over red feel so distressed by hostile emotions? Being able to express angry feelings is as essential to healthy emotional development as the capacity for displaying love and compassion.

What makes the 'green over yellow' child so concerned about revealing his or her joy? Perhaps there is a belief that happiness is a dangerous emotion to reveal because it inspires jealousy or irritation in others. Such anxieties are not uncommon in children whose parents lack a sense of humour and take an over-serious view of life.

Six
Exploring Your Child's Anxieties

Once you are satisfied that anxiety is at the bottom of your child's problems, proceed to Step Two and try to gain a general idea of what's causing the problems. Some children are afraid of so many things that it is hard to know where to begin. They are shy at school, fearful with friends, withdrawn at home. Almost everything seems to make them anxious. Others, like Max with his exam nerves or Sally with her spider phobia, can face up to almost any challenge except in that one area where they cannot cope at all.

Even when you are fairly sure of what is causing your child's fears, it's worthwhile carrying out a detailed assessment. If you simply tackle what seems to be the cause of the problem, but is only a symptom of it, you will fail to banish your child's anxiety.

You may recall, for instance, that although Max's anxieties focused on examinations, they actually stemmed from a belief that God was punishing him for being 'sexually perverted'. This false belief needed to be identified and eliminated before his exam nerves could be successfully overcome.

As you will have realised, studying your child's pictures and drawings not only helps to identify anxiety as being responsible for difficulties, but often provides helpful clues as to the reasons for those anxieties. The recurrence of particular themes, for instance, offers a good insight into a child's anxious preoccupations.

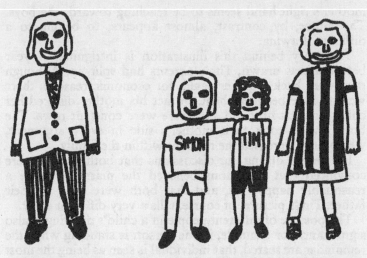

Another way of using pictures to identify areas of anxiety is by asking your child to draw himself or herself in different situations which you suspect may be causing difficulties, at school, playing with friends, with brothers or sisters and so on. There is no need for any artistic skills, since stick people are perfectly satisfactory indicators.

Study the finished picture carefully and notice whether there are any differences in size between the figures. Has he, for example, drawn himself much larger or smaller than other people depicted? Where children are shown playing, how has your child drawn herself? Joining in with the others or standing isolated and alone at the fringes of the group?

When the whole family have been portrayed, who is shown standing closest to the child? Physical distance in a drawing is usually an indication of emotional closeness or separation in real life. Has she placed herself closer to her father or her mother, to an older or younger brother or sister? Is she part of the group, or remote from them?

In the picture above, nine-year-old Tim has drawn himself, with his parents and ten-year-old brother Simon. Notice how the father has been placed at a distance from the rest of the family. The closeness between these three is emphasised by the way Simon is resting on Tim's shoulder, while his mother's right hand seems to be reaching towards the boys. The father, by contrast, almost appears, to belong to a different drawing.

The story behind this illustration is intriguing. A year before it was drawn, Tim's parents had split up. Although they were back together again, for economic reasons, there was no love between them. In fact his mother disliked her cold, sarcastic husband and there were constant rows. The boys always took their mother's side in every argument, which only increased the tensions within the family.

It emerged during our discussions that both parents were convinced that their sons believed the marriage to be a reasonably happy one, and that both were fond of their father. Tim's picture, of course, tells a very different story.

The posture of different people in a child's drawing is also significant. For example, if one person is standing while the remainder are seated, that individual is seen as being the most dominant member of the group.

Here, Richard aged nine, has shown his father standing and clearly giving orders while the rest of the family sit and listen. During our interview he admitted being frightened of his father, who was very critical of his son's behaviour.

When looking at your child's drawings, probe for general areas of anxiety by asking:

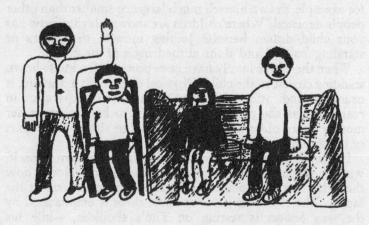

'What are the people in the picture doing?'
'What are they saying?'
'What are they most likely to be doing next?'
'What they are most likely to be saying next?'
Your child's answers to these questions can provide valuable insights into the nature of anxieties and fears.

A picture assessment

Now I'll show you a way of identifying specific anxieties through a series of illustrations showing one day in the life of a child called Dibs. This is known as a *projective* test, since it works through your child projecting anxieties on to the character in the strip. It is designed to look for major causes of anxiety in younger school-age children (6 to 14) and comes in two parts The first is a series of questions for your child to answer, the second a questionnaire about your child for you to answer.

Part One

This tells the story of what happened to Dibs on his first day back at school. I have made Dibs a boy, because experience has shown that girls are more willing to identify with a boy character than boys are with a girl. At the same time, the drawings have been made in such a way as not to suggest either sex especially strongly. It is for the same reason that the name Dibs was chosen.

The idea behind the assessment is that your child identifies with Dibs, and, by deciding which way he would be most likely to respond in the situation described, projects his or her own anxieties on to the character. If you are reading the story aloud to a young child, it is perfectly all right to use a more familiar name, although you must avoid using his or her own name, that of a relative or a close friend. Should you do so your child may respond in the way he or she knows that familiar individual would react.

When reading aloud you may also wish to change some of the words in order to make the meaning clearer. This is permissible so long as the meaning is not altered. When reading aloud, be careful not to suggest which alternative you favour by emphasis, expression or tone of voice. The exercise takes around fifteen minutes to complete and should be done in a single session.

Dibs goes to school. This is a story about Dibs and what he did on his first day back at school after the summer holidays. When I was writing about Dibs, I wasn't sure what he would have said or done. Please help finish the story. Here's what you must do. Beside each picture you'll find a choice of two things Dibs might have thought, or said, or done.

Decide which of the two you think is most likely and write the letter on a separate sheet of paper. There are no right or wrong answers, so you cannot make a mistake. Just put yourself in Dib's place and make your choice.

1

Dibs woke up on the first day of term to find the sun shining brightly through his bedroom window. Then he remembered that the holidays were over. This made him feel:

a: pleased at the thought of meeting his friends again;
b: miserable because he hated school.

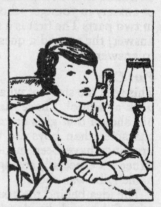

2

When Dibs had washed and dressed he went down to the kitchen where his mother was cooking breakfast. She wanted to know if he was looking forward to school and Dibs said he was because:

a: he was excited to be starting a new term; b: he didn't want his mother to know how unhappy he felt.

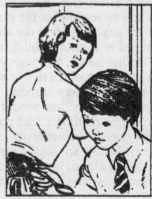

3
While walking to school, he saw a group of boys from his class. Dibs:

a: went over to them and chatted, then they all walked on together; **b:** did not join them because he felt too shy.

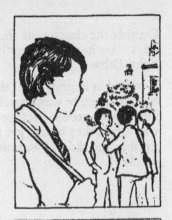

4
As he approached the school gates, Dibs was thinking about all the new subjects which he would be studying that year and wondered:

a: if he would find them interesting; **b:** how well he would be able to understand them.

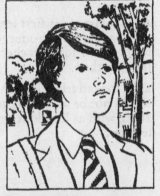

5
Going through the school gates, Dibs noticed a new boy standing all by himself. He:

a: strolled over and chatted to him; **b:** felt sorry for the boy because he looked lonely, but did not feel like chatting to him.

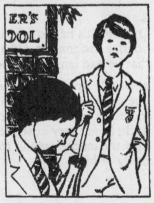

6
Outside the classrooms some boys were having a friendly fight. Dibs:

a: joined in happily until the bell sounded; **b:** went quickly into the classroom because he was afraid they would get into trouble and did not want to be involved.

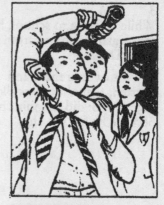

7
At the start of his first lesson, the headmaster introduced them to their new form teacher. Dibs thought that:

a: he looked friendly; **b:** he would not be as easy to get along with as his old form teacher.

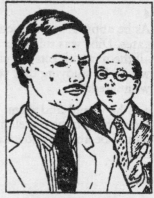

8
Opening his bag to take out his holiday assignment, Dibs found that he had left it at home. He:

a: wasn't worried because he knew the teacher wouldn't be too cross with him the first day back; **b:** felt very upset because now the teacher would think badly of him.

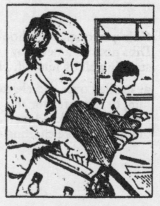

9

The new teacher read out their timetable. As he spoke, Dibs, thought that it:

a: sounded more interesting than last term's timetable; **b:** was fearful that he would do badly in many of the new subjects.

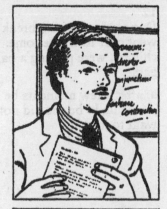

10

The teacher asked for a volunteer to collect the new textbooks from the stores. Dibs immediately put up his hand because:

a: it was a chance to get out of class for a while; **b:** he wanted the teacher to think well of him.

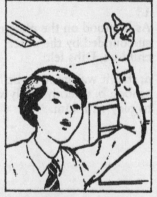

11

Later that morning, Dibs was working on some problems when the teacher came and looked over is shoulder. This made Dibs:

a: work even harder; **b:** become confused because he felt sure the teacher was going to criticise his answers.

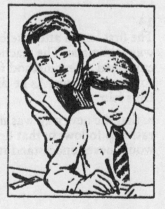

12
During the morning break, Dibs
went over to where some
children were playing a ball
game:

a: after a few moments he
joined in; **b:** but he did not
want to join in.

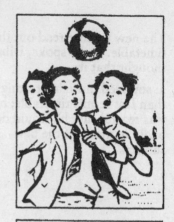

13
As he stood on the playground
surrounded by the other
children, Dibs felt:

a: that it was good to be back at
school; **b:** nobody really wanted
to play with him.

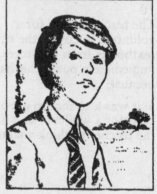

14
The first lesson after the break
was arithmetic. The teacher
explained a new method for
solving problems. As he did so,
Dibs felt:

a: that the new way was much
easier to follow; **b:** that he
would never understand it.

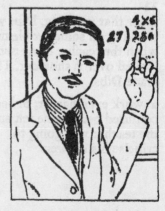

15
As they started working through sample problems, Dibs noticed that the boy beside him was getting different answers. He immediately thought:

a: the other boy didn't know what he was doing; **b:** that he was the one who didn't understand and was making mistakes.

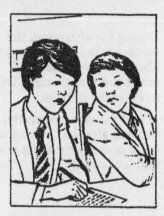

16
At lunch most of Dibs' friends went into the canteen to eat. But he:

a: ate sandwiches he had brought from home; **b:** didn't feel like eating because he was too unhappy.

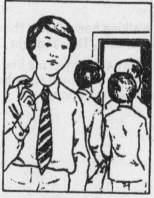

17
Dibs sat down in the sunshine, closed his eyes and started to daydream. In his imagination he:

a: saw himself playing with his friends on the beach and having a great time; **b:** was back home with his mother and would never have to go to school again.

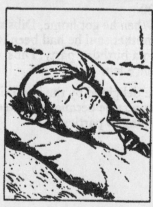

18
During the afternoon, the
teacher asked them questions
about the work they had
studied in the morning. Dibs
knew many of them:

a: and answered correctly; **b:**
but was afraid of putting up his
hand in case he made a mistake
and looked silly.

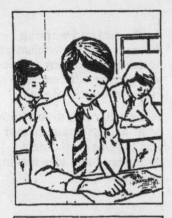

19
Walking home from school that
afternoon, Dibs thought that:

a: he had enjoyed his first day
back; **b:** he would soon be
safely back home.

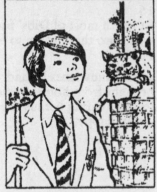

20
When he got home, Dibs's
mother said he had been invited
to a birthday party. Dibs at
once felt:

a: delighted by the invitation; **b:**
miserable because he hated
going to parties.

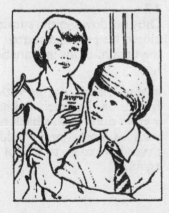

Part Two

You should complete this portion of the assessment based on how your child has been behaving over the past few months. Make a note of any of the statements which apply on a separate sheet of paper. Avoid marking the book because you may wish to repeat the assessment in a few months' time to check on progress.

My child:

1 becomes moody and/or miserable during the last few days of the school holiday
2 seldom brings home friends from school
3 stays close to my side and rarely explores alone when we visit anywhere new
4 always tries very hard to please
5 doesn't like starting a new leisure activity
6 plays alone much of the time
7 is more prone to minor ailments during term time
8 is very obedient
9 doesn't enjoy going to parties
10 needs a lot of encouragement from adults
11 is reluctant to tackle an unfamiliar challenge
12 cries a lot when school starts
13 finds it hard to make new friends
14 sets great store by praise from grown-ups
15 is upset by changes in routine
16 is made miserable by one or more school subjects
17 takes more time than most to settle into new surroundings when we go on holiday
18 becomes upset if even mildly criticised
19 seldom seems to join in games with other children
20 is often in a black mood on returning from school
21 wets the bed occasionally
22 has nightmares fairly regularly
23 often finds it hard to fall asleep
24 has a poor appetite
25 bursts into tears for no apparent reason
26 is generally fearful
27 is often irritable or aggressive
28 clings to me when away from home

29 gets very upset if scolded
30 has more than four colds a year

How to score

Part One
To score Dibs's diary, ignore all **a** responses. Award one point for every **b** chosen.

Part Two
Award one point for each statement with which you agreed.

Now total the points for Parts One and Two as shown in the table below.

Pictures and statement		Total points
1: Anxiety over going to school		
Pictures:	1, 16, 17, 18, 19	
Statements:	1, 7, 12, 16, 20	
2: Anxiety over making friends		
Pictures:	3, 5, 12, 13, 20	
Statements:	2, 6, 9, 13, 19	
3: Anxiety over meeting expectations		
Pictures:	2, 6, 8, 10, 11	
Statements:	4, 8, 10, 14, 18	
4: Anxiety over anything new or unfamiliar		
Pictures:	4, 7, 9, 14, 15	
Statements:	3, 5, 11, 15, 17	
5: Physical signs of anxiety		
Statements:	21, 22, 23, 24, 25, 26, 27, 28, 29, 30	

When you have totalled the scores in each of these five areas separately, add them all together to produce a further score for the whole assessment. Now use both the individual and total scores to identify the comments, below, which apply to your child.

What the assessments reveal

Total score for Parts One and Two less than or equal to 12
Your child does not, at present, appear to be suffering from unhelpfully high levels of overall anxiety in his life. It could still be, however, that specific situations, activities or individuals produce a sufficiently high increase in anxiety to undermine your child's intellectual performance or emotional health.

Four areas of life were anxiety is especially likely to occur in childhood are:

* Going to school.
* Making friends.
* Living up to expectations.
* Coping with novel or unfamiliar challenges.

These were explored in the pictures and statements grouped together in the assessments, and are considered in more detail below.

It is also important to appreciate that changes in your child's lifestyle may radically increase levels of anxiety. For example, transferring to a new school, or even to a different form, a change of teachers, the break-up of a close friendship and moving to a new neighbourhood can all adversely affect anxiety.

Children who were previously coping well at school or at home may fairly rapidly develop the sort of emotional and behavioural problems associated with feeling excessively anxious. Events capable of producing such changes are not always recognised by parents as of special significance in their child's life.

Because anxiety can arise at any time, keep a watch on your child's anxiety levels – especially during periods of change – both by observing changes in emotional state and behaviour, and the confidence with which certain challenges are met. You will also find it useful to follow the procedures described in later chapters for managing anxiety and stress.

Total score for Parts One and Two 13–20
A score in this range suggests that there are certain situations, activities or people which make your child unhelpfully anxious. The level of anxiety is not, at the moment, excessive and should not be causing any major problems.

However, if the total was achieved by a high score in just one of the assessment areas, it is still possible that your child has an anxiety problem in that particular sphere of life. If allowed to continue it could undermine motivation and cause lasting damage to self-esteem. The specific areas where such anxiety may be occurring are considered below.

Total score for Parts One and Two 21–29
The score obtained suggests that your child may be experiencing unhelpfully high levels of anxiety in certain areas of life. These are considered in detail below. It is important to start working with your child to reduce his or her anxieties in the area of greatest concern.

Total score for Parts One and Two greater than 30
This high score suggests that your child is currently experiencing a serious anxiety problem in several areas of his or her life. Read the comments under the relevant headings below, and then start using the practical procedures described in the chapters which follow to combat those anxieties. If allowed to continue unchecked they will not only make it very hard for your child to achieve his or her true potential, but could also lead to health problems and emotional difficulties.

Now look at your child's scores in each of the five areas. These examined anxieties specific to:

• Going to school.
• Making friends.
• Meeting expectations.
• Coping with anything new or unfamiliar.

In addition, physical signs of anxiety were examined.

Going to school: score 4 or less
(Pictures: 1, 16, 17, 18, 19. Statements: 1, 7, 12, 16, 20.)
Your child does not appear to be experiencing any great
anxiety over school in general, although it may well be that
a specific subject, a particular teacher, difficulties in
adjusting socially or some other aspect of school life is
proving troublesome.

You may have noticed that increased anxiety, perhaps
resulting in tearfulness, a reluctance to go to school or even
feeling physically ill, occurs on particular days of the week. If
this is the case then use the *positive listening* procedure
described in Chapter Seven in order to help you pinpoint the
specific cause of such problems.

Going to school: score 5 or more
This type of anxiety is quite common and could be caused by
concern over a single subject or the attitude of a particular
teacher. Equally, it may be caused by a general inability to
cope with the intellectual challenges of school, dislike of
routine or clashes with authority in general. It may also be
due not so much to anxieties about attending school as
worries over what may be happening at home while he or she
is away. This is most likely if your marriage is going through
difficulties, if you are moving home, there is sickness in the
house or trouble with another child.

Making friends: score 4 or less
(Pictures: 3, 5, 12, 13, 20. Statements: 2, 6, 9, 13, 19.) Your
child does not seem to be experiencing any excessive anxiety
over social situations. Friendships are being made and
sustained without significant difficulty.

Making friends: score 5 or more
A high score here suggests that your child finds it hard to
make friends or handle social situations. This could be due to
a recent change of schools, or moving to a higher form and
leaving his friends behind. There may also be a more deep-
seated problem underlying his anxiety.

Children who do especially well in class often feel isolated from the rest of their companions because they have so few interests in common. Nursery-school children who learn to speak earlier than most, for instance, find it much easier and more interesting to make friends with adults than infants of their own age.

However, it is important for children to acquire the skills needed to make friends and be generally sociable with others of a near age.

Meeting expectations: score 4 or less

(Pictures: 2, 6, 8, 10, 11. Statements: 4, 8, 10, 14, 18.) Your child does not appear especially concerned about gaining the approval of adults. To some extent this is a healthier attitude than excessive dependence on the approval of parents and teachers. If taken to extremes, however, a total absence of anxiety over satisfying adult expectations can undermine motivation and so impair intellectual performance.

It may be that he is insufficiently motivated where specific subjects are concerned. Children sometimes adopt apathy as a means of protecting themselves against distressing anxiety. Once we have stopped caring about an outcome there is little cause to feel anxious about it.

Meeting expectations: score 5 or more

Your child appears to be over concerned about satisfying adult expectations and meeting the many demands which he sees as being imposed by this need. While it is essential for children to feel that parents and teachers are concerned for them and want them to do well, too much anxiety can lead to a loss of confidence, an over self-critical and self-blaming attitude, decline in motivation and a negative self-image.

The child who strives mainly for adult approval and praise will become over influenced by the opinions of others. This leads to an emotional dependency that can be damaging to intellectual growth.

Your child must develop confidence in his own ideas, judgements and decisions. He must also learn to accept the consequences of inevitable mistakes and failures without becoming excessively distressed.

Coping with anything new or unfamiliar: score 4 or less
(Pictures: 4, 7, 9, 14, 15. Statements: 3, 5, 11, 15, 17.) Your child does not appear especially anxious in unfamiliar situations or when faced with novelty. This is extremely useful, since successful intellectual development depends on a willingness to tackle new challenges and experiment with situations not previously encountered.

Sometimes, however, the total absence of anxiety in the presence of a novel event stems from a lack of interest in what is happening.

Coping with anything new or unfamiliar: score 5 or more
Your child seems to be made anxious by the need to tackle any new or novel tasks. This may lead to a desire to avoid anything unfamiliar. When avoidance becomes a regular part of your child's response to the threat of novelty intellectual and emotional growth is stunted.

It is important for children to exercise their curiosity and acquire the skills which can only be mastered by experiencing a wide range of new situations, activities, places, people and so on. Achievement often demands the assurance to venture into uncharted territory, experiment with different ideas and seek fresh ways of tackling problems. In all these activities the child made over fearful by novelty will be severely handicapped.

Physical signs of anxiety: score on statements 21–30: 1–2
The few behaviour problems you have noticed are caused by anxiety. Although not severe at present, it will be helpful to reduce the underlying anxieties by using the procedures I describe in later chapters.

Emotional outbursts, disturbed sleep, poor appetite, and even bed wetting, are best treated as symptoms of anxiety rather than problems to be dealt with in isolation.

Physical signs of anxiety: score on statements 21–30: 3 or more
The problems which you have observed in your child are rooted in excessive anxiety. These symptoms can occur even where the score on the Anxiety Assessment is not especially high.

However much you may be irritated by, or disapprove of, your child's behaviour recognise that he or she may be as distressed by it as you are. These problems are best tackled at their roots by identifying and helping resolve underlying difficulties.

Now that you have a good general idea of the areas of life which are causing your child anxiety, the final step can be taken. You must pinpoint the precise situations, activities and circumstances that pose the problems.

Seven
Pinpointing Specific Anxieties

Now you have a general idea of the area in which to search for your child's anxiety. The final step is to identify the specific cause responsible for these difficulties. The only person who can give you this information is, of course, your own child. And the only way that knowledge may be gained is by empathic listening.

Are you a good listerner?

When you are busy or distracted, it is all too easy to listen to a child without hearing what is being said. In fact, research has shown that parents pay attention to less than a quarter of all the things children tell them. When it comes to discovering the specific source of your child's anxieties and fears, attentive listening, so that you hear what is left unspoken as well as the words actually said, is essential.

There are five golden rules for being a good listener.

Never do two things at once

You are busy cooking lunch when your youngster comes rushing in with something urgent to say. At such times it is all too easy to fall into the trap of distracted listening. You hear with half an ear instead of paying attention. The only way to avoid this is by assigning priorities to the tasks in hand.

If cooking is more important, tell your child in a firm, but friendly, way that you just aren't able to stop and listen properly at that moment. Then arrange a time when you can give her your undivided attention. Don't worry that this will discourage or upset her. Most children feel flattered that you are taking their ideas seriously enough to spend time on them.

If you sense that your child has something to tell you that is more vital than carrying on with lunch, then stop what you are doing, sit down and listen carefully.

Don't listen when upset

Strong emotions – anxiety, anger, disgust, guilt and so on – filter out all but a small part of what your child is trying to tell you. It is human nature to pay the most attention to information which supports a view we have already taken. For instance, you have come to the firm conclusion that your child has been very naughty. As he attempts to explain his conduct, anger gets in the way of your attending to what is said. Instead, your emotions magnify any remarks which justify the rage you feel.

When Tony brought home a bad school report, his father was furious. Convinced that his son had been lazy, Martin was in no mood to pay attention to the eight-year-old's tearful explanation of conflicts with a new teacher which had made him fearful. As a result, Martin not only failed to discover what had caused the poor report, but his son is very reluctant to ask him for help again.

Never attempt to listen until you have calmed down and are capable of assessing the situation objectively.

Don't be dismissive

Ten-year-old Jane begged to have the hall light left on as she dropped off to sleep. Her mother considered this babyish nonsense. 'You walk home from school in the dark,' she pointed out. 'I know I do,' explained Jane. 'But that's different. Darkness feels more scary indoors.'

This intriguing comment revealed some deeply rooted

anxieties about what was going on at home. Had her mother listened attentively, she might have used this to start a discussion about Jane's feelings on a whole range of subjects. But, having made up her mind that her daughter was talking nonsense, she dismissed the child's explanation even as it was being made. 'Don't be so silly,' she said curtly, clicking out the light.

Listen positively

This means paying attention and listening with your eyes as well as ears. Set aside time so that you can devote your full attention to what is being said. For younger children, those few moments when they've been tucked up in bed can be an ideal time for such a discussion.

In one family I know, mother and daughter have a nightly 'me time', during which they discuss all that has gone on during the day. Even when nothing has happened to make the child anxious, 'me time' provides a wonderful opportunity for setting the happenings of the day in perspective.

If probing for anxieties, start the conversation with a friendly but neutral remark such as, 'You seem a bit upset today. Would you like to talk about it?' Once your child starts talking, you should speak as little as possible. Encourage his or her disclosures through the use of body language, by nodding, smiling and showing obvious interest.

You may have noticed that this is how experienced television chat-show hosts encourage their guests to talk. Professional training has taught them that an unnecessary word or comment can disrupt the speaker's train of thought or cause them to clam up. So they nod, smile, look interested and give a great deal of silent encouragement for the other person to keep talking. And, when probing an especially sensitive topic, they are not afraid of silences. Instead of rushing to fill the void with unnecessary words, as we so often do in everyday conversation, they allow the person time to collect his thoughts or gather her courage to make some painful admission.

Even if the things your child is saying make you upset, keep those feelings to yourself – at least for the time being.

Your expression must remain friendly, your comments encouraging and sympathetic. The appropriate time to express hurt, anger or disapproval is after you've listened long enough and carefully enough to understand what's gone wrong. Any interruptions, especially critical comments, will only inhibit self-disclosures and make it impossible for you to get to the heart of the anxiety problem.

Pay special attention to your child's tone of voice. Does he sound miserable when telling you something which, on the face of it, seems to be good news? A conflict between what is being said and how the words are spoken will often provide clues to painful emotions simmering below the surface. Be alert for self-mocking comments like: 'I'm just too weedy to stand up for myself . . . I'm too dumb to understand that . . . Dad's always saying I'm a clown.' Even when self-mockery is wrapped up as a jest, or uttered with a smile, it may be expressing ideas or feelings which arouse great anxiety.

Observe facial expression, gestures and posture. Physical tension in the face, hands, or body betrays an inner stress. Fidgeting, playing with a pencil or pen, pulling at the lobe of an ear, scratching the nose or cheek are all signs of carefully suppressed anxiety.

Be aware of pauses, hesitations or repetitions in your child's flow of talk. These can be caused by conflicts between what is being said and what your child would really like to say. Slips of the tongue can be equally revealing. Freud believed that such slips, known technically as parapraxes, were highly revealing of inner tensions.

When one fifteen-year-old girl client described her mother as being : 'all *fright*' instead of 'all right', it was a revealing slip since the woman was very well-meaning but perpetually nervous.

Incidentally, the word parapraxis can also be used to describe these occasions when your child 'accidentally' loses some urgently needed item. For example, Mike, aged nine, was always leaving his bathing costume behind on school swimming days. He was also terrified of water. It's likely that this 'forgetfulness', while not a deliberate ploy to avoid having to swim, was unconsciously motivated by his fear of the pool.

Positive listening is not easy. It take patience and practice to get it right. There is often an overwhelming desire to comment on an error of fact, offer reassurance when your child admits to a fear, or criticise an irritating admission. Yet such interruptions only make it harder to find out what's really going wrong.

Adopt the approach of a good GP trying to diagnose a patient's ailments by listening to the description of symptoms and watching out for signs. If, each time the patient said anything, the doctor jumped in with a remark or condemnation, very little progress would be made. Suppose, when the patient admitted to smoking heavily, the GP sneered sarcastically: 'What a fool you are! How can I help anybody so deliberately self-destructive?'

Is it likely that any further confessions would be made? Almost certainly the patient would clam up about any other life-threatening habits for fear of attracting further criticism.

Encourage your child to talk freely by saying little but listening attentively. Don't be afraid of silences and rush to fill them with words. Give your child space to think, to reflect and to summon up the courage to make an admission which he or she is fearful will upset you.

If the conversation really does seem to have ground to a halt, try rephrasing and repeating back the last comment your child made. This demonstrates that you've been paying attention, clarifies your understanding of her comment and allows her to view the remark more objectively. For example, your child might explain miserably, 'I hate Mallen, he's always picking on me. He loathes me . . .'

If no further explanation is forthcoming, and it appears that he's lost for words, try saying quietly, 'I understand. Mr Mallen doesn't like you and picks on you.'

Your child may then continue. If not, ask a question related to the last complaint: 'How does he pick on you?' or 'What kind of things does he say or do?'

Always try to get specific examples of behaviour or activities which are upsetting your child. It's impossible to remove anxiety when the causes are vague and tenuous. For instance, if all you get out of your child is that she's afraid of a particular teacher because she's 'cruel', there is no way of knowing what form her cruelty takes, or whether it really is 'cruel' at all. She might, for instance, simply refuse to allow your child to play around as freely as a more easy-going teacher.

Ask for examples and don't be fobbed off with imprecise accusations. If your child is incapable of telling you just why a particular activity or person causes him or her to be anxious, there may well be a deeper layer of difficulties to be uncovered.

One eight-year-old boy complained how beastly his stepfather was and how much better he treated his older brother. But he was unable to provide any examples of his stepfather's supposed dislike of him, or describe ways in which he favoured the brother. All he could say, with increasing irritation, was: 'Well, he does . . . he does hate me.'

The anxiety here was not caused by anything his stepfather said or did – in fact, the man was extremely kind to the boy – but arose from anxiety about men in general. He had never forgiven his natural father for deserting them two years earlier.

Do not try and make notes when your child is talking, since this will only undermine the relaxed atmosphere essential for success in positive listening. Instead of a friendly chat, your child may see it as more of a formal interrogation. I suggest that you pay close attention to what is said and then make a brief note of comments and ideas immediately after your discussion. Some parents use a tape-recorder to capture the whole conversation. How successful this proves depends on your child's feelings about being recorded. But never do this secretly, since it would rightly be seen by your child as a flagrant breach of trust.

You have now identified the general areas in which difficulties are occurring, and pinpointed the specific situations, activities or people responsible for making your child anxious. But before you start to create a programme for dealing with those anxieties you need to take one further step – which is to explore your own anxieties.

Eight
Discovering Your Own Anxieties

In order to help your child overcome his or her anxieties it is important to understand your own feelings and fears. Parents who are generally anxious, or have a phobia, often ask whether their children are at risk of 'catching' such fears from them. In the sense that your child might 'catch' a cold of flu bug the answer is no, but there are still three ways in which such anxieties can be, and often are, passed on to your child.

The first is through your genetic structure – that biochemical blueprint, passed from parents to their children, which determines such things as height, body build, skin pigmentation, eye colouring and so on. There is evidence that when one or both parents have above-average anxiety, their child may be born with a natural predisposition to feeling more anxious than his or her companions.

What happens is that the sympathetic branch of the ANS (see Chapter Three) is especially sensitive to arousal and thus more readily triggered in such youngsters – and, once turned on, it is harder to bring under control. This inborn tendency to fearfulness is called *trait* anxiety, in contrast to *state* anxiety, which means being afraid of external circumstances.

It is a matter of everyday experience that some people approach life more timidly and apprehensively than others. Such individuals are regarded as having a more introverted personality than the bold, seemingly nerveless, extroverts who throw themselves without hesitation into any number of challenging situations.

The positive side of being born with this sensitive type of ANS is that it seems to be associated with faster and more efficient learning. Provided that they learn to manage their anxieties, so as not to be panicked and overwhelmed by them, such children tend to do better in school. A less happy aspect of their ability to learn very rapidly is that they are probably more prone to develop phobias. As we shall see in Chapter Fourteen, a single scary experience, with say a dog, a cat or a spider, may be sufficient to produce a phobic response in these especially vulnerable people.

Because trait anxiety is inborn there is nothing you can do to remove it. You can, however, teach children powerful procedures for controlling their 'step-up' mechanisms. By doing so you enable them to use a potentially damaging predisposition to maximum advantage in any challenging situation.

The second way of passing anxieties to your child is through the process known as 'modelling'. It is seldom appreciated just how much of what children learn about life is acquired by simply watching other people's behaviour and then copying them. Any parent with two or more children knows only too well how imitative brothers and sisters can be. If the older child messes around with his food or plays with a particular toy, the younger one immediately wants to copy him. Accents and manners are an especially good example of modelling in action. A child may speak and behave quite differently at home than she does at school. Modelling teaches your child how he or she is expected to behave in a wide variety of situations. Indeed, most of what we know results from observing and modelling.

Unfortunately, adult anxieties and phobias can be passed on to the child through exactly the same process. If, for instance, you are terrified of spiders there is a far better chance of your child also developing such a fear, although not necessarily to the same extent.

The third method by which your own anxieties can affect your child is through the defence mechanisms you use to protect yourself against such anxiety. Let's look, for instance, at the widely used strategy of avoidance. Here is how the interplay of anxieties might occur.

Your child is fearful and unhappy at school. Her distress, quite naturally, makes you upset and slightly anxious. To protect yourself you avoid the issue. Rather than listening to her difficulties and taking whatever practical steps might be needed to make life easier, you avoid discussing the matter.

Or you may use denial of reality, by insisting that things aren't as bad as she claims. 'Don't be silly, darling,' you tell her reassuringly. 'You'll soon settle down and enjoy it.'

You could also use the defence of rationalisation, comforting yourself with the thought that, 'Every child is unhappy at school, it's all a part of growing up.'

There may, of course, be a certain amount of truth in such assumptions, which is why they can work so well as defensive strategies. The problem is that, by lulling you into a false sense of security, they prevent you from confronting and dealing with a situation in its early stages. This often means that a difficulty which might have been fairly easily resolved when it first started can develop into a major problem which is far harder to resolve. Furthermore, your apparent indifference to the child's distress makes him or her feel even more misunderstood and abandoned.

You may recall that Max, the teenager with excessive anxiety about taking examinations, believed he was being punished for perfectly normal and natural sexual behaviour. On the one occasion when, fearfully and tentatively, he began to broach the true nature of this fear to his mother she immediately shut up like a clam and refused to discuss the matter further. 'I don't want to listen to anything like that,' she told him angrily.

Her own problems and anxieties in coming to terms with sex meant that she immediately resorted to avoidance, and denial of reality, when confronted with the topic. There are many, many other anxieties which adults have with regard to their children that can cause similar barriers to discussion. The seven most common, in my experience, are:

- Homosexuality. Any discussion of same-sex attraction frequently arouses extreme anxiety in parents.

- Relationships with people considered unsuitable on the grounds of social class, background, race or religion.
- Inability to achieve goals which the parent has set for the child.
- Refusal to follow pathway in life planned by parents. For instance, they want her to become a doctor, she's determined to be an actress. He wants to be a dancer, his parents have always dreamed of his becoming a lawyer.
- Rejection of parental beliefs, whether religious, social or political.
- Need for greater independence, especially in the early teens.
- Any behaviour considered dishonest, such as lying, stealing, truancy etc.

If you have specially strong views in any of these areas, or are made very anxious when contemplating them, it is going to prove extremely difficult for you to help your child deal adequately with his or her own anxieties. Unless you are able to adopt a relaxed and objective attitude towards discussing such issues, which does not necessarily mean you have to endorse them, attempts to assist could end in disaster. Your child might become even more anxious and, just as bad, further alienated from you. In such situations it is often better for another member of the family, who does not find it difficult to talk about the subject in a neutral manner, to offer the assistance.

In many cases, however, these problems can only be avoided by understanding, and then coming to terms with, your own anxieties – and then learning how to bring them under control. By comparing your anxieties with those of your child it is also possible to identify some of the ways in which you may be adversely influencing him or her.

Assessing your own anxieties

Like all assessments which ask you to choose between two responses, you may find some of the statements below tricky and frustrating to answer. You might feel that your actual response would depend on things like your mood, who was with you, what else was happening and so on.

This is inevitable in such an assessment and will not

invalidate it, provided that you respond rapidly without giving yourself pause for thought. An immediate response is most likely to be an accurate reflection of your subconscious, emotional reaction to the statement. If this doesn't seem to work and you find yourself stuck for an answer, think back to a similar situation within the past six to twelve months. Reflect on how you felt or behaved at that time.

1 A party invitation from people I know only slightly makes me feel: **a**: pleased at the chance of getting to know them better; **b**: unhappy at the prospect of meeting relative strangers.

2 If asked to tackle an unfamiliar activity, I am most likely to: **a**: agree readily and feel reasonably confident about measuring up to the challenge; **b**: try to avoid it but, if unable to do so, approach the task with little confidence of success.

3 When somebody I am fond of says or does something I consider unwise, I am most likely to: **a**: make my views known; **b**: stay silent for fear that my criticism will harm our relationship.

4 On waking, my first thoughts are most likely to focus on: **a**: the jobs to be done during day; **b**: apprehension over what the day will bring.

5 If somebody pushed ahead of me in a queue, I would probably: **a**: point out that I was ahead of them and insist on keeping my place; **b**: say nothing for fear of causing a scene.

6 If invited to join a local club or society, my immediate response would be to: **a**: consider the suggestion seriously; **b**: feel sure I would not enjoy it.

7 When given a deadline for a complicated task, I feel: **a**: a new sense of urgency and energy; **b**: panic that I cannot finish in time.

8 Most of the time I feel: **a**: confident of my ability to deal with life's challenges; **b**: overwhelmed by life's problems and difficulties.

9 I have little difficulty making new friends: **a**: true all or most of the time; **b**: rarely true.

10 When I have finished some task I am: **a**: interested to know

what my partner or colleagues think about it; **b**: concerned that others will criticise my work.

11 If invited out to dinner by new friends, I: **a**: look forward to the invitation; **b**: worry about not making a favourable impression.

12 If I noticed people staring at me when I was out in public, I would assume that: **a**: I must be looking especially attractive; **b**: something was wrong with my appearance.

13 If given instructions which I do not completely understand, I am most likely to: **a**: seek clarification; **b**: hope for the best rather than appear foolish by not understanding.

14 If faced with the prospect of spending an evening alone, I would: **a**: be pleased by an unexpected invitation from a friend; **b**: resent missing a chance of being on my own.

15 If offered advice over a tricky task in which I have expertise, my usual response is to: **a**: assume that I know best; **b**: immediately believe the other person must be right.

16 When I make a mistake in a complicated task, I will usually: **a**: sort out the error with little or no loss of confidence; **b**: feel thrown by the blunder and find it hard to regain my lost confidence.

17 If watched while performing a task by someone more expert than myself, I: **a**: carry on without feeling stressed; **b**: find myself making silly mistakes out of anxiety.

18 I feel fearful of what the future may hold for me: **a**: rarely or never; **b**: fairly frequently.

19 I think people who plan their futures are: **a**: sensible, because we must all prepare for tomorrow; **b**: deluding themselves because one can never know what's going to happen next.

20 When arranging my summer holidays I: **a**: eagerly anticipate the fun it will bring; **b**: find myself worrying about what could go wrong.

How to score

The only responses of interest are the **b** statements. Total these, then refer to the charts below to discover the extent to which anxiety is affecting your performance and may be influencing your child.

Total number of Bs	Level of anxiety
15 + (*high*)	You appear to be generally over-anxious and find many situations difficult to cope with.
9–14 (*medium*)	Pay special attention to those situations which cause special anxiety (see below).
1–8 (*low*)	This level of anxiety should not be causing you any general problems. But there could still be specific areas of difficulty (see below).

As well as assessing your overall anxiety level, the questionnaire examined your responses in the same four areas of life as we explored for your child. This enables you to discover whether similar anxieties are shared. If they are, it is especially important to learn to control such anxieties in yourself, to avoid adversely influencing your child and provide him, or her, with the most effective help.

Your child's score 5 or more on the statements below	Your own score 3 or more on the statements below	Area of anxiety causing most difficulty
Pictures: 1, 16, 17, 18, 19 Statements:		School/Life in general
1, 7, 12, 16, 20	4, 8, 18, 19, 20	Includes: coping with demands, worry over the future, fears about what may go wrong.

Your child's score 5 or more on the statements below	Your own score 3 or more on the statements below	Area of anxiety causing most difficulty
Pictures: 3, 5, 12, 13, 20 Statements: 2, 6, 9, 13, 19	1, 6, 9, 11, 14	Social anxiety Includes: meeting people, making friends, getting on with others.
Pictures: 2, 6, 8, 10, 11 Statements: 4, 8, 10, 14, 18	3, 5, 10, 12, 17	Expectations anxiety Includes: making a good impression, being needed, being loved, having a good reputation.
Pictures: 4, 7, 9, 14, 15 Statements: 3, 5, 11, 15, 17	2, 7, 13, 15, 16	Novelty anxiety Includes: tackling anything new or unfamiliar, acquiring skills, or knowledge.

If you both scored above average on a particular area of anxiety, it is probable that your child is, at least to some extent, following your example in being made anxious by – and possibly attempting to avoid – activities which come under that heading.

If this is the case you should work together to reduce such anxieties. How this may be done I shall be explaining in the chapters which follow.

Part Three
Banishing your child's anxieties

Nine
How To Help Your Anxious Child

While all children feel anxious or fearful at some time in their lives, no child ever experiences these feelings for exactly the same reason or in precisely the same way – which is why there can never be a neatly defined approach to helping your child overcome anxiety and fear. To be successful the plan you adopt must take into account both your child's unique view of the world and his or her individual circumstances.

This means not just exploring your child's response to different situations, but also seeing how his or her response affects others. There is a constant, dynamic interplay between the way one person feels, thinks and acts and the way in which others respond to them. This response in turn influences the first individual's thoughts, emotions and actions. In the example below, anxiety has caused a child to behave in a particular way, which influences her mother's responses. Observing these responses, the child alters her own behaviour, thereby changing that of the mother – and so on.

To see this interplay at work, let's imagine a first meeting between five-year-old Mark and his new teacher. The small boy's anxiety over starting school makes him shy, diffident and unresponsive.

The teacher observes this behaviour and decides that Mark needs reassurance. She kneels down, holds his hands and talks quietly to him. Mark observes her behaviour and starts feeling less anxious. He smiles and begins answering her questions. Seeing him become less anxious and more confident, the teacher decides that it is time to give attention to other children. He observes her walking away and starts looking miserable again. She notices this and comes back.

As you can see, the boy and the teacher produce important changes in one another's behaviour by the way they behave.

Child	Teacher
Thinks I can't cope.	
Feels Anxiety.	
Behaves Looks scared.	
Cries.	
	Observes
	Thinks He's afraid.
	Feels Sympathy.
	Behaves Cuddles and
	talks reassuringly.
	Smiles.
Observes	
Thinks It's going to be OK.	
Feels Less scared.	
Behaves Stops crying and	
looks less fearful.	
	Observes
	Thinks He's not so
	anxious now.
	Feels Less concerned.
	Behaves Stops
	cuddling.
Observes	
Thinks I'm on my own again.	
Feels Scared again.	
Behaves Looks anxious and	
fearful	
	And so on . . .

When developing a programme to help your child defeat handicapping anxiety, phobias and fears, it is important to take this constant interplay into account. Everything you say or do to your child when helping her manage anxiety will have an effect on the way she thinks, feels and behaves. Her behaviour is going to change not only your own thoughts, feelings and actions but also those of your partner and your child's brothers and sisters, friends, teachers, fellow pupils and so on. So let's consider the different influences on your child and the extent to which such an interplay occurs. These are illustrated below:

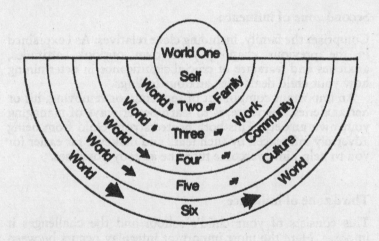

First zone of influence
At the centre is your child and his or her self-image. Here the interplay between behaviour and feelings is especially powerful. As he carries out different activities, a child observes himself and his emotions.

For example, when struggling with a maths test, the child feels increasingly anxious over his failure to understand the questions. The negative thoughts aroused by this anxiety increase tensions in his body. He notices his heart beating more rapidly, his mouth growing dry, his tummy churning, and so on. This deepens panicky thoughts, undermines confidence and reduces motivation to continue. Performance declines still further, leading to a further rise in physical arousal, even more unhelpful thoughts and handicapping emotions.

In order to deal with this aspect of anxiety your child must be taught practical procedures for controlling mental and physical feelings. In addition, he or she must be helped to adopt a more positive and constructive attitude towards any challenges currently arousing unhelpfully high levels of arousal.

Second zone of influence

Comprises the family, including close relatives. As I explained in the previous chapter, your own outlook, attitudes, anxieties and fears are of crucial significance in determining how your child deals with anxious feelings.

An important component of reducing, or removing, his or her anxieties, therefore, is to learn better ways of managing your own anxiety. This both protects your child from being adversely influenced by such fears and makes it far easier for you to help him overcome those he already possesses.

Third zone of influence

This consists of your child's school and the challenges it imposes. Here the most important interplay occurs between your child and his or her teachers. Although usually less powerful than the influence of parents and children, the effect of these exchanges is potentially even more significant because teachers have so much power to affect a child's future.

There are various ways of reducing anxiety over school activities. Some involve teaching your child new skills to increase motivation or enhance self-esteem. Others require the assistance of the school in bringing about the changes required. The best methods of approaching school-based fears and anxieties are fully described in Chapter Eleven.

Fourth zone of influence

This is your child's life away from school and the friends he makes, or fails to make. Here too there are many practical steps which can be taken to reduce anxieties, and I shall be discussing these in Chapter Fifteen.

Fifth zone of influence

Finally, there are the influences exerted by society and the world at large. These include such potential sources of anxiety as violence, on TV and in real life, and worries about unemployment, illness and nuclear war. As we saw in the second chapter, these are of significant concern to a majority of teenagers.

Here the need is to help your child handle such threats in a mature and realistic way. How this may be done is described in later chapters.

Phobic fears

These arise within the first sphere of influence, since they are entirely due to the way in which an individual perceives the world. But they can be triggered by people, objects, activities or situations which may arise in any of the remaining four spheres: in the home, at school, in your child's social life or in the world in general.

Depending on their nature and duration, phobias can often be removed without too much difficulty, provided that the appropriate procedures are used. I shall explain how these are best dealt with in Chapter Fourteen.

Summary of the anxiety antidote

This is a practical, self-help plan which enables you to help your child deal with anxiety, phobias or fears arising in any of the spheres or influence. The general features of this plan are:

• Teaching your child, and yourself, procedures for managing the physical and mental symptoms of anxiety.

- Teaching your child, and yourself, ways of developing a positive, confident attitude towards anything which now creates unhelpfully high levels of anxiety.
- Showing your child mental skills, such as better ways of revising for examinations, that will prevent anxiety from arising in the first instance.
- Making such changes as are necessary, and possible, in your child's surroundings in order to eliminate sources of needless anxiety and stress.

Ten

The Relaxation Response

Toddlers, drunks and professional athletes have one thing in common – they can take heavy tumbles without hurting themselves. A small child stumbles over his feet and falls to the carpet; there may be tears of rage but there are unlikely to be any broken bones. Similarly, a drunken man can take a fall which, when sober, might break an arm or leg, yet escape unscathed. A skier may lose control on the slopes, then spin and tumble through the snow for hundreds of feet before slithering to a halt, bruised and shaken but not in need of plaster casts.

In each case the absence of serious injuries is a result of the same thing – complete physical relaxation. The toddler was relaxed because infants have not yet learned to be needlessly tense, the drunk because of the sedating effects of alcohol on his brain, and the athlete because of rigorous professional training.

Such cases are, however, the exception. Most people, most of the time, are far from relaxed. From the age of three or four onwards we start tensing up our muscles, not just deliberately, in order to use them, but unknowingly and unintentionally as a result of anxiety. In the end, unnecessarily stressing certain groups of muscles – especially those of the face and neck – becomes such a habit that we are not even aware of the resulting tension. Just as families who live alongside railway lines stop noticing the noise of passing trains, so we rapidly cease paying attention to the distress signals from our muscles.

The results are greater vulnerability to emotional stress and to such unpleasant physical problems as back pain, leg cramps, stiff shoulders, or neck- and headaches.

Noticing normally hidden tensions

As you sit or lie reading this book, pause and focus on your muscles. Some of them – those holding the book, for example – you have tensed voluntarily. But what about those which are not doing the work of supporting the book, turning pages or holding your body in a certain posture – are these needlessly tense?

Start by paying attention to the muscles of your forehead and jaw. Do you notice any tension there? Now frown hard. Really tighten up your forehead while, at the same time, clenching your teeth tightly together. Hold this tension for a count to 5. Let go. Smooth out the furrows in your brow and let your lower jaw hang loose. Notice the difference between tension and relaxation.

Next, focus on your neck muscles, shoulders and back, and see whether any, or all, are tensed. Repeat the exercise by deliberately tightening these muscles. Shrug your shoulders hard and, at the same time, press your head against the chair. Hold the tension for a count to 5, then relax. Let your shoulders sag and your head loll back against the supporting chair.

By tensing and relaxing muscles you not only make it easier to detect unnecessary tensions, but also to eliminate them. These two exercises are part of a very effective relaxation procedure which I shall describe in more detail later in this chapter. Suitable for both adults and children, it brings about a very deep state of bodily relaxation.

Almost everybody carries around with them the burden of needless tensions. By becoming more aware of this problem, and teaching your child to notice when he or she starts growing tense, you are well on your way to bringing anxiety under control.

Children get tense too

It is sometimes difficult for parents to accept that children as young as four or five can experience high levels of unnecessary muscular tension. As they grow older these problems generally become worse, and by their early teens as many as six out of ten children suffer from some form of stress-related problem.

The relaxation reponse

Relaxation is the body's natural antidote to anxiety. It strengthens the *parasympathetic*, or slow-down branch of the ANS (see page 30), while combating the effects of the *sympathetic* or step-up component. As a result it helps regulate such signs of anxiety as rapid heart rate, uneven breathing, increased sweating, dry mouth and churning stomach.

With the bodily feelings brought under control, it is far easier to banish the negative mental responses, feelings of panic and the sense that things are getting out of control.

In the first part of this home-help plan, I am going to describe three ways of relaxing, the first two suitable for young children, generally under the age of 8, and the third for older children and adults.

Teaching your child to relax

Most children enjoy being taught relaxation techniques so long as they are presented to them in the right way and the sessions are seen as a sort of a game. You are most likely to attract their interest and sustain motivation by following these six simple rules.

1 Keep the atmosphere friendly. Never put pressure on your child to carry out a particular exercise since, by doing so, you will only increase anxiety – thus defeating the whole purpose of the training.
2 Never give the impression that the training is some kind of punishment or a sign that you are annoyed with them. It should be presented as something to look forward to and enjoy.

3 When your child does well, be sure to offer praise and encouragement. But don't be critical if he or she has difficulty in carrying out a particular part of the training.
4 Select a time of day when you can devote all your attention to the session and go through it unhurriedly. Avoid intruding on your child's play time or favourite TV programme.
5 Choose a quiet room. If you have other children not going through the training, exclude them from the room during these sessions to avoid making the child feel self-conscious. Take the phone off the hook and hang a 'do not disturb' sign on the door.
6 Sell the training to a reluctant child by explaining the benefits of relaxation in terms of their favourite leisure time pursuit – playing a sport, athletics, dancing, riding, gymnastics or chess.

You can explain, quite truthfully, that many top athletes, dancers, horsemen and chess grand masters use similar procedures to prepare themselves mentally and physically for major contests. The US Olympic ski-team, for example, have long used relaxation and mental imagery (a procedure I shall describe later in this chapter) to enhance their performance on the slopes. So too do international marksmen, sprinters, high-jumpers, boxers and fencers. You can reassure any boy who feels embarrassed or uncomfortable about this training that it is in no way sissy.

If your child is more interested in intellectual pursuits, you can explain that these procedures will make it possible to learn things more quickly, understand things more easily and achieve greater success during tests, examinations or any other mentally demanding activity.

The essential thing is to develop your child's interest and confidence in these procedures so that they will be used automatically and unselfconsciously whenever the need arises. Read the instructions a number of times, so that you have a good grasp of them, before embarking on the first training session.

The room
This should be comfortably warm and, preferably, carpeted. If it is not give your child a soft rug to lie on. For the second

of these exercises you also need some bouncy, lively music for your child to jump around to. A cassette tape is easier to use than a record since you are going to be stopping and starting the music several times.

What to wear
Loose-fitting clothes, such as a track- or jump-suit. No shoes should be worn, but keep socks on to prevent feet from getting cold.

Time of day
Not immediately after a large meal, as your child is too likely to fall asleep, or when he is over-tired. Just before normal bedtime is good, and helps promote deep, restful sleep. Keep the sessions fairly short, fifteen minutes at the most.

Relaxation training for the under-eights
(The age is only approximate. Some mature eight-year-olds may prefer the adult relaxation procedures. Equally, there are children of nine and ten who still enjoy the more playful approach of the first two procedures.)

Most young children can learn to relax quickly and easily once they have been taught to identify, and release, unnecessary muscle tensions. The approach consists of giving your child some vigorous exercises to do, described below, either in real life or in the imagination, designed to *increase* muscular tensions. You then draw your child's attention to the feelings in his muscles and encourage him to unwind each in turn.

When your child is physically relaxed, you present him with various drawings – Floppy Bear, Fearless Tiger or Happy Hound (see the illustrations on pages 130, 132, 134) – which will intensify feelings of relaxation, confidence or happiness. This pairing of images and emotions helps your child to switch quickly to a positive frame of mind in real-life situations. By associating Floppy Bear with relaxation, for instance, your child develops the ability to relax at will simply by bringing an image of the bear to mind. These techniques will be described in more detail later in the chapter.

Relaxation Method One: Active imagination
Start by asking your child to sit down in a comfortable chair, lie back and close her eyes. Now ask your child to imagine any vigorous activity, one that demands a great expenditure of energy, such as: racing to the cinema so as not to miss the start of an exciting film; dashing home to see their favourite television programme; running a race on school sports day, and managing to win by inches; chasing after the last bus home or sprinting to catch a train that will take them down to the seaside.

Talk your child through the scene, adding excitement by keeping your voice lively and using a rapid rate of delivery. At the end of the session, he must flop down and feel all the tension easing out of his muscles as it would do if he really was resting after some exhausting action. Young children usually have no difficulty in picturing such a scene in their mind's eye, so long as you provide many of the details.

After a few moments spent imagining the hectic activity, bring it to an end. Your child breasts the winning tape, then flings herself, panting with exertion, on to the grass. Or he jumps aboard the bus or train and drops thankfully into his seat.

Now direct your child's attention to his legs, arms, shoulders and torso. Tell him to imagine that his limbs are feeling warm, heavy and floppy. His eyes should remain closed and his breathing should be light and even. Pick up one arm and, if there is any tension, tell him to let go and allow the arm to flop, so that it becomes limp in your grasp. Slowly and gently lower it to his side. Now repeat with the second arm. Tell him to feel his body sinking more and more deeply into the chair.

These instructions, following the imagined burst of activity, will help him notice and banish needless muscular tensions and so make him feel more and more deeply relaxed.

To see how this exercise goes, let's eavesdrop on Marian and seven-year-old Tamsin.

After they both sit down in comfortable chairs, Marian explains that they are going to play a game.

Marian: 'I want you to imagine you are going to the seaside for the day. You have to catch a train. If you miss it you may not get to the seaside in time for a swim . . . Oh, look, I can see the train pulling into the station. Quick, we shall have to run. Run . . . run . . . run . . . Listen, I think the guard's blowing his whistle. Run as fast as you can . . . open the carriage door . . . plop down on the seat. How do you feel after running so hard?'

Tamsin: 'Puffed out . . .'

Marian: 'How would it feel if I lifted one of your arms?'

Tamsin: 'Floppy . . .'

Playing in the imagination works well for many children, who love to fantasise about winning races or catching the train to the seaside.

Other youngsters learn more rapidly if the activity takes place in real life rather than in their mind's eye. For these children, the Puppet Dance is more suitable.

Relaxation Method Two: *The puppet dance*

You explain to your child that he or she is a puppet, with strings attached to head, hands and feet. Here's Marian taking Tamsin through the Puppet Dance. After explaining how the strings have been attached she says: 'When I pull this string your arm is going to come up.'

She makes a lifting movement above Tamsin's right hand, and the little girl obediently raises her arm. 'Now this one and your left leg comes up. When I pull this one your head comes up. I want you to dance around like a puppet as I pull the strings.'

At this point, play some music and allow your child to dance around as you pretend to pull on the strings. After a little while say something along these lines: 'Now I'm going to pull on one of the strings as hard as I can.'

Marian pretends to tug on the string attached to Tamsin's right hand, and the little girl's arm jerks obediently up. 'I'm pulling as hard as I can, higher and higher . . .'

Entering enthusiastically into the game, Tamsin raises her right arm as high as she can manage.

'Now I'm going to cut the string . . . here come the scissors . . . there goes the string.'

I suggest that you make a cutting gesture with two fingers, slicing through the strings one by one. Dramatise the moment at which your child should drop an arm or a leg and allow it to go completely floppy.

With all the strings cut, your child drops to the carpet or on to a comfortable chair. Now, as before, lift each limb in turn and, if they are not fully relaxed, encourage her to let them flop into your hands. Remember that your child should lie still, have her eyes lightly closed, and keep breathing lightly but evenly.

Emphasise the increasing bodily relaxation with comments like: 'Your legs are getting heavier and heavier . . . your arms feel heavy, and warm, and floppy. Feel yourself sinking more and more deeply into the chair.'

This method is especially good for active children who need to burn up some energy in order to relax at all. If tensions remain after the first dance, 'reattach' the strings and repeat. This can be done several times, with each cutting of the string leaving your child feeling more and more deeply relaxed.

Relaxation Method Three: Muscle-focusing
This procedure is suitable for adults and older children. It consists of focusing on each of the major muscle groups in turn.

First, each group of muscles is deliberately put under tension, as you may have done above when I asked you to tense your forehead and jaw muscles, then release them. This simple action rapidly trains the mind to notice the difference between needless tensions and a state of relaxation in all the muscles. You will need to practise for fifteen to twenty minutes a day for around fourteen days to master the procedure. But, once learned, it may be used to reduce the symptoms of physical anxiety in many situations.

You can practise at any time of the day, although if you do so just before bedtime it will help you enjoy a better night's rest. The only snag is that either you or your child may drop off to sleep before completing the session. If this happens regularly, switch to the morning or early afternoon, although you will still find it beneficial to relax again immediately before going to sleep.

You, or your child, may prefer to relax in a dimmed room, perhaps with some soothing background music. Sitting in an easy chair, or lying on a couch, bed or the floor are equally satisfactory and simply a matter of personal preference. At first you may like to experiment with different approaches until you find the one with which you or your child feels most comfortable. Shoes should be removed, and any tight clothing undone. Legs must be uncrossed, hands resting by your sides.

Read through the instructions below a few times so that you are familiar with them and no longer need the book to guide you. If you want to relax with your child, why not make a tape-recording of the instructions and play it back as you sit, or lie, side-by-side going through the movements?

To remember the order in which muscles are to be first tensed and then relaxed use this memory jogger: *A Soothing Feeling – Totally At Peace*. The first letter of each word identifies the key muscle groups involved.

A = Arms and hands.
S = Shoulders and neck.
F = Face (forehead, jaw, tongue, eyebrows).
T = Torso (chest and stomach).
A = Ankles, legs and buttocks.
P = Pictures which help to intensify the feeling of
    relaxation or enhance some other positive
    emotions.

First close your eyes lightly, rest your head against the chair or bed, flop out your arms and let your legs go limp. Keep your breathing light and regular. Each time you exhale say the world CALM silently to yourself and imagine all your tensions flowing away from your body with the expelled air. Take some moments to practise breathing and repeating CALM on each exhaled breath. Next:

Arms and hands. Form your hands into fists, and clench them as tightly as possible. While doing so, try and touch your shoulders with the back of your wrists. Feel the tension building up. Hold it for a slow count to 5. Let go completely, allowing your hands to rest beside you and feel all the tension flowing down your arms and out of your fingertips, disappearing into the room, never to be seen again.

While tensing the muscles in your hands and arms, notice if any other muscles also tighten up; for instance, when clenching your fists, see whether your jaw or forehead becomes more tense. We often place several unrelated sets of muscles under tension simultaneously, a bad habit which makes it far harder to perform efficiently.

For instance, if your child has learned to tense his hand and jaw muscles together, clenching his fist while answering a question in class could make it impossible for him to speak clearly. Should you notice, or your child comment on, such related tensions, make a special note of them. By breaking the connection you automatically reduce tension elsewhere in the body. Next:

Shoulders and neck: Turn your attention to the muscles in your own, or your child's, shoulders and neck. Since these muscles usually contain much needless tension, tackle the different groups one after the other.

To tense your neck muscles, press back against the support on which you are sitting or lying. As before, increase the tension, feeling it building up in the muscles, then hold for a slow count to 5. Relax and let your head rest lightly back against the support. Your breathing must remain regular and, on each exhaled breath, the word CALM is silently repeated.

Tense the shoulder muscles by hunching them as hard as possible. Raise the shoulders upwards. Higher . . . higher . . . Hold for a slow count to 5. Drop your shoulders and feel them flop. Notice any tensions flowing away from neck and shoulders, and intensify this sensation by imagining them being expelled from these muscles each time you breath out. Next:

The face. You tense jaw and tongue muscles by clenching the teeth while pressing the tip of your tongue against the roof of the mouth. Clench tightly . . . tighter. Press hard . . . harder. Hold for the same slow count to 5. Relax. Let go. Allow the tongue to lie loose in the mouth, parting your jaws slightly. Repeat the word CALM each time you breathe out and, with every expelled breath, notice tensions flowing from jaw and tongue, down the arms and away from your body through the fingertips.

Eyes – deliberately tense these muscles by screwing your eyes tightly shut. Press the lids together firmly . . . hold for the same slow count to 5. At the same time, frown as hard as you can. Relax again. Unwind the muscles, allowing the eyelids to rest lightly together and the brow to smooth right out. Notice, or instruct your child to notice, the difference between tension and relaxation in these muscles. Next:

The torso. Tense the chest and stomach muscles by taking a very deep breath. Draw the air far into the lungs until your chest seems incapable of expanding any further. While doing this, flatten the stomach muscles by drawing the tummy in towards the spine. Tell your child to try and 'touch' his backbone with his belly-button. Hold for the same slow count to 5. Breath out fully and allow the stomach muscles to relax. Feel tensions draining away from the body, leaving behind a feeling of deep peace and calm.

No tensions in the hands and arms.

No tensions in the shoulders and face.

No tensions in the chest and stomach.

Ankles, legs and buttocks. Tense all these muscles by stretching the legs, pointing the toes and squeezing the buttocks tightly together. Hold for a slow count to 5 before allowing the legs to relax completely. Feel the tension streaming out through your toes and vanishing into the room, leaving you feeling very deeply relaxed. Carry on breathing quietly and lightly and repeating the word CALM with each exhaled breath, and then go on to the next stage.

Creating a mind movie

By teaching your child one of the three physical relaxation exercises I have described, you will be providing him or her with a powerful antidote to the physical symptoms of anxiety. Any time he or she starts feeling anxious, or just before some stressful challenge – such as taking an examination – ten minutes spent relaxing the muscles will help keep unhelpful tension under control.

But there is one additional skill you need to teach. I call this creating a Mind Movie, because it involves developing a powerful mental image. There are three important reasons for doing so.

Firstly, it is not always convenient to go through any of the three procedures described above, since these take time and need somewhere private and quiet to carry them out. If your child is suddenly confronted with a test in class, for instance, she can hardly disappear for ten minutes in order to relax. But by linking a specific image to a feeling of relaxation, and then deepening the sensation by using an additional technique which I shall describe in a moment, your child will be able to banish tensions quickly and without anybody else noticing what is going on. It is the perfect antidote to anxiety in a hundred and one situations where any other kind of relaxation procedure would prove impossible.

The second reason for creating Mind Movies is that, while muscle relaxation strengthens the slow-down branch of the ANS, so making your child more resistant to anxiety, it does not entirely still the mind. Indeed, research in my laboratory has shown that people can be deeply physically relaxed, yet have extremely agitated minds. Unless both brain and body are in an equally calm and controlled state, anxiety can still wreak havoc with performance. Using Mind Movies is a way of focusing, calming and soothing the brain, thus enhancing its ability to resist negative and anxiety-arousing thoughts.

Finally, we shall be using the same procedures for helping your child deal with anxiety in specific situations, such as answering questions in class, playing a sport, meeting people for the first time and combating phobic fears.

I will start by explaining how to create a soothing image in your own mind, or that of an older child.

Island of peace

After completing a relaxation session, and banishing physical tensions from each of the main muscle groups, remain sitting or lying. Focus on your breathing for a few moments, and each time you exhale feel yourself becoming more and more deeply relaxed.

In your mind's eye, transport yourself to a desert island. If teaching this skill to your child, describe the island in sufficient detail for him or her to conjure up a suitable image, but not so precisely that there is no scope for personal imaginings. This must be a very personal place, where your child feels entirely at ease.

See a sunny beach of golden sand. A crescent-shaped bay, perhaps, fringed by palms and tropical flowers on one side and by the clear blue waters of a tropical ocean on the other. You are lying on the sand feeling warm, comfortable, safe and secure. On every side there is beauty: blue skies, a golden sun shining down, soft sand and a calm sea lapping the golden beach. This is your own special place, a haven to which you can return any time you start to feel stressed, tense or anxious.

Imagine, or encourage your child to imagine, the scene as vividly as possible. In this Movie there is not only colour and sound, but also smell – the smell of tropical blossoms and touch – the warmth of the sun and sand. Listen to small waves uncurling and retreating. Taste a cooling fruit drink. You are relaxed and at peace. There is no tension, no anxious thoughts to disturb your mind.

Spend several minutes in that haven. Breathe lightly, and silently repeat the world CALM each time you breathe out. Imagine that, as the waves flow away from the beach, they take with them the last of your anxieties. Focus on these feelings and enjoy them. You are at peace with yourself.

Freed from stress.

Freed from tension.

Freed from anxiety.

You feel warm, contented and secure.

Now, place the first two fingers of each hand on your forehead, just above each eyebrow. Take your child's hand to direct his fingers to these spots. You should easily find two small areas of raised bone, slight bulges beneath the skin. These are pressure points used in Japanese massage to induce relaxation. Lightly press down on these bumps with your fingertips and, while doing so, repeat to yourself: 'I need only do this to feel relaxed and confident.' Massage the bumps lightly for a few seconds while repeating that instruction. Then let your hands rest

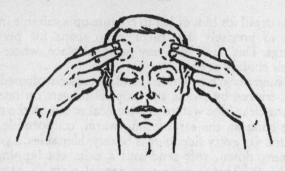

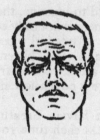
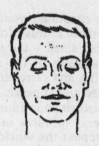

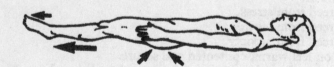

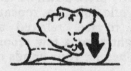
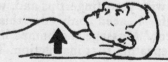

at your sides and spend a while enjoying the feelings of relaxation and contentment.

To return your child to the world, count slowly backwards from 5 to 1. When you reach 1, tell him to open his eyes and get up slowly – too fast a movement and he may feel slightly giddy. Instruct him to go about his next task calmly, while trying to preserve the feelings of relaxation.

In describing a desert island for the Mind Movie, I am not suggesting that it is the only image which will prove successful in stilling anxious thoughts. Many people find the island helpful, but others prefer to create their own scenes. Some like to picture themselves lying in the grass of a sunny meadow, listening to a nearby stream and smelling the scent of wild flowers. Another popular image is being curled up in a comfortable armchair, by a blazing log fire, while the rain beats against the windows.

The precise content of the image is unimportant. All that matters is that the person directing the Mind Movie feels very calm, relaxed and secure.

Two common difficulties

At the start of training, you or your child may encounter two common difficulties. The first is a sudden increase in tension immediately after the relaxation starts taking effect. If this happens don't worry. It is perfectly normal and will disappear with continued practice. What happens is that, as we start to let go of the anxiety habit and notice tensions leaving the muscles, part of the brain gets scared by the notion of letting go. Unconsciously we fear the consequences of losing control, and this switches on the step-up branch of the ANS, increasing sympathetic arousal and making us feel more tense than before.

The second difficulty is an inability to concentrate. Your child might find that, as he starts to conjure up his Mind Movie, distracting thoughts or worries come flooding in and destroy the images. Again this is quite usual and vanishes with further training. If there is an especially persistent and distracting thought, one of these strategies may prove helpful.

Tell your child to imagine the worrying idea written on a sheet of paper which is then tossed into a fire. As it burns and vanishes in a cloud of smoke, so too does the worry. Alternatively, the worry could be spelled out in sand at the edge of the tide. The sea comes in and washes away both the words and the anxiety. A similar method is to ask your child to imagine writing this concern in chalk on the school blackboard, and then wiping it clean. Any image which allows him first to express the anxiety, and then have it destroyed in some way, could prove beneficial.

Rapid relaxation

After practising regularly for a couple of weeks, simply picturing the relaxing scene (while briefly fingertip-massaging those two trigger points on the forehead) will be sufficient to produce deep feelings of mental and physical relaxation. Your child can use this any time he or she wants to relax and calm down quickly without attracting attention.

Using Floppy Bear – helps relaxation

This is a method for linking a relaxing image to a state of deep physical relaxation in younger children. Because they

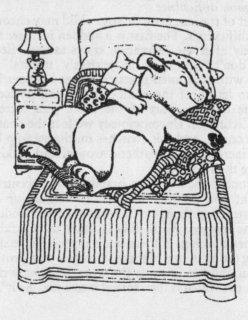

usually find it very hard to create or sustain the kind of Mind Movie which proves so effective with adults and older children, we need to adopt a different strategy.

This is where the picture of Floppy Bear comes in useful. Here's how to use him.

Go through either *Active Imagination* or the *Puppet Game* to relax your child's body. Now, as she lies back in the chair, or stretches out on the floor, ask her to recall any occasion when she felt snug, comfortable and safe. Perhaps it was tucked up warm in her own bed, or snuggled close to you on a sofa in front of the fire. Encourage her to talk about this scene, describe it to you and to recapture the good feelings which it produced. When she has done so, show her the picture of Floppy Bear and say something along these lines:

'I want you to look at the picture of this old bear. His name is Floppy Bear. See, his arms and legs are all floppy. He's going to help us to remember that the first thing we do each morning is relax. And, any time you start feeling frightened, all you've got to do is think about Floppy Bear and he'll make you feel better.'

If Floppy Bear appeals to your child, you might suggest that he or she traces it out of the book to produce a colour picture that can be pinned up in the bedroom. One of the first things your child sees on waking up will then be this relaxation-inducing image. In this way your child is encouraged to stay relaxed while starting the day.

If your child has a favourite doll or cartoon character which is more familiar or better liked than Floppy Bear, you may prefer to use this instead. The important thing is to teach your child to associate a certain image with a relaxed mental and physical state. After a number of practice sessions, just conjuring up the image of Floppy Bear (or whatever) will make your child feel less anxious and tense.

Here's how the mother of seven-year-old Alex described the way Floppy Bear helped her son cope with school anxieties created by an unpleasant teacher.

'Alex said that when he started his work in the mornings he felt his heart "thud-thudding" when the teacher stopped at them all, and he panicked and it stopped him working even more, so we introduced Floppy Bear after the relaxation and also did the Puppet Dance each day before school. Alex's own comments after about one week. "When I feel the worry starting, I think of Floppy Bear and I just get on with the work and before I know I'm finished."'

Using Fearless Tiger – builds confidence

You can use the Fearless Tiger picture in much the same way as Floppy Bear, only this time to boost a timid child's confidence – for example, when being teased.

As with Floppy Bear, the best time to introduce this character is immediately after a relaxation session. This time, ask your child to think of some occasion when he or she was feeling very confident and in control of the situation. One eleven-year-old remembered how confident he felt when speeding around the park on his brand-new red and silver skateboard. An eight-year-old girl recalled her positive

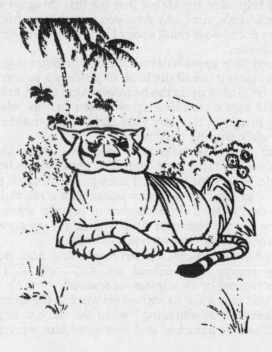

feelings when doing gymnastics. The precise situation is unimportant; all that matters is that it should inspire your child with a belief in himself or herself.

Ask your child to bring that activity to mind as vividly as possible. Then show him Fearless Tiger and explain that, just by thinking of the Tiger, he'll give his confidence a boost. If your child likes the Tiger picture it can also be traced from the book, coloured and pinned up in a prominent place in his bedroom. On waking each morning he can look at the Tiger and top up his confidence for the day. Again, if there is a character which also symbolises being confident and in control, such as Superman, to which your child relates more easily, use this in the same way.

Using Happy Hound – increases joy

Even when a child has learned to control his anxiety in a certain situation, he may not derive much pleasure from it – even when the activity is supposed to be enjoyable. For example, a child who is very shy about meeting strangers should, with your help, be able to cope with going to a party. But while all the other children are laughing and having a good time, he could be left isolated by his lack of enjoyment.

Use Happy Hound to help improve matters in exactly the same way as Floppy Bear and Fearless Tiger. Here you ask your child to remember an occasion when she felt very happy, perhaps during a visit to the pantomime, zoo or when going on holiday.

Help develop these positive emotions by discussing how pleased and excited she was at the time. Then, when she is feeling happy, show her the picture of Happy Hound and explain that, if ever she feels miserable, bringing him to mind will help make her happier. As with the other characters, you can replace Happy Hound with any other cheerful image, such as Mickey Mouse. If the Hound finds favour with your child, however, he too can be traced and coloured for display in the bedroom.

It is important to work at developing all these positive emotions – don't expect them to emerge instantly. The images will only start triggering relaxation, confidence or happiness

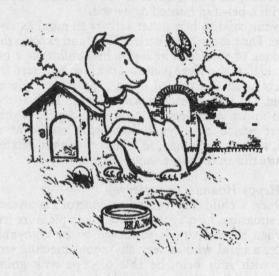

after being associated with those feelings after a relaxation session on several training sessions.

In teaching your child how to relax, mentally and physically, and by helping improve his or her emotional response to stressful situations, you will provide powerful techniques for managing anxiety. Sometimes this is all that will be needed to solve the problem.

When approaching previously anxiety-arousing situations in a more relaxed and positive manner, your child will find it possible to cope well with situations which previously caused considerable distress. Furthermore, his or her performance in other challenging activities – such as playing sports, taking exams, making new friends and so on – will also be enhanced.

This greater mastery creates greater motivation and builds self-esteem. Instead of being trapped in a negative spiral, where poor performance leads to increased anxiety, thus undermining performance still further, you will have helped

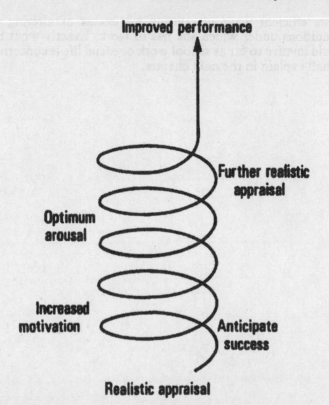

Improved performance

Further realistic appraisal

Optimum arousal

Increased motivation

Anticipate success

Realistic appraisal

to develop the positive cycle illustrated above.

This time your child views his chances of success realistically and tackles the task with confidence. He is able to put any setbacks into perspective more easily, and be less discouraged by inevitable mistakes. His level of arousal remains at optimum for undertaking that activity – an important point which I shall be discussing in more detail in the next chapter.

There will also be occasions, however, when providing your child with these anxiety-management procedures is not sufficient fully to overcome his or her difficulties. In this case it will be necessary to try and bring about changes in other areas. This may mean teaching her additional skills, such as more efficient ways of revising for exams or altering the conditions under which she has to work. Exactly what this could involve so far as school work or social life is concerned, I shall explain in the next chapter.

Part Four
Helping with
specific anxieties

Eleven

Helping Your Child With School Anxiety

The child whose first few weeks at school are made as happy as possible is less likely to become the victim of anxiety later on. This is true whether he or she is starting school for the first time, or moving to a new school. There are four main sources of anxiety when your child starts school. With a little planning all can be made less alarming and far easier to cope with.

1: Anxiety about the unknown

On my first day at primary school, a teacher asked me to go and ring the bell for break. I left the classroom and looked around for the bell push. Seeing what looked like the right button, I pressed it firmly. The next instant, classroom doors were flung open as children raced into the playground. I had set off the fire alarm!

You can probably remember a similar horror story, perhaps of being told to go to the cloakroom, or a particular classroom, and having not the slightest idea which direction to head. Tell your child frankly that things are going to seem strange and a bit frightening. Explain that he will probably get lost, not know where to sit, to hang his coat or wash his hands – but that nobody will mind him asking.

Although the first few days at school are usually taken up with showing children where everything is located, there can be so much information to take in that your child easily becomes confused. If possible, take him to the school before terms starts. Let him meet his form teacher and look around the building to get an idea of where things are. Some primary schools arrange for new pupils to come along before the beginning of term in order to meet their teachers and learn the lay-out of the buildings. This is an excellent idea, and you should always take advantage of such opportunities. Even when the school does not organise such visits, however, the head teacher is usually willing to show parents and new pupils around, provided that arrangements are made well in advance.

2: Anxiety over following rules

Your child may find that doing something you allow at home gets her into trouble with the teacher. On the other hand, things you forbid, such as playing around with sand and water on the table, may be encouraged. Conflicting rules and regulations can cause anxiety and confusion at first. So too can having to follow a timetable and do things according to the clock rather than their own personal whim. Following school discipline becomes far easier if your child has been firmly, but fairly, disciplined at home. Have a minimum of rules – too many may restrict intellectual and emotional development – but apply them consistently.

3: Anxiety over activies

These include dressing and undressing to go to the lavatory, or for games, gym, dancing or swimming. Make sure your child's clothes are easy to take off and put back on again; many small children simply cannot cope with laces, buttons or ties. If compelled to do so, especially under the gaze of an impatient teacher, they can become extremely anxious – and even less capable. Use slip-on shoes, ties with elastic bands that can be slipped under the collar, and elasticated plimsoles.

4: Anxiety over separation

Merely being away from you may make your child extremely anxious at first, but as she settles down and forms an attachment to her teacher another problem can arise. This is a conflict between love for you and loyalty to her teacher. If you disagree with the teacher openly, and in front of your child, she may start to become very anxious. Whom should she side with – the mother she adores or the teacher she has grown to like and respect? If you do have an issue to take up with your child's teacher, therefore, do so out of earshot of your child.

Because so many anxiety problems could be avoided, or more easily eliminated, if there were good lines of communication between home and school, it is useful to know how to talk to teachers. Unfortunately, while this sounds simple, a great deal can go wrong.

Talking to your child's teachers

Talking to teachers can leave the most self-assured adult suddenly feeling five years old again. A flood of old memories makes it hard to have an adult conversation. Instead, there's a tendency to revert to childlike behaviour. Depending on your personality, you could find yourself becoming either submissive and deferential or bossy and domineering.

Needless to say, neither approach helps open those lines of honest conversation so essential for helping your child overcome, or avoid, school anxieties. Here are some suggestions for making such exchanges more pleasant and productive:

1 Attend as many open days and PTA meetings as possible. Get to know your child's main teacher informally; both of you will feel easier and less defensive when talking to a familiar face than to a remote stranger.

2 Make certain of all your facts before you complain. The most truthful child can misunderstand or misinterpret a situation and there is considerable temptation for children to exaggerate in order to make their complaints seem more reasonable.

Jean was furious when her nine-year-old, Susan, was kept

behind after school to complete a homework project she had failed to hand in on time. Susan insisted that the work was not due for at least another week. Jean's first reaction was to confront the teacher with the seemingly unfair treatment handed out to her daughter, but before embarking on a confrontation she was sensible enough to double-check the facts. A phone call to another mother revealed that Susan was mistaken about the deadline, and the teacher had been well within her rights to punish her.

3 Never say or do anything while angry. Rather than dashing straight to the school, phone for an appointment. Explain calmly, and concisely, the reason for your complaint and arrange a mutually convenient time to discuss it.

4 Plan your questions and the desired outcome before the meeting. What do you want to find out? What do you hope to achieve from the discussion? If you feel uncertain about remembering key facts, make a brief written note and do not worry about reading from it during the meeting.

Never worry about being branded a 'troublemaker' or making life harder for your child by your complaints. Provided that the approach is courteous and constructive, good teachers will welcome your interest and involvement.

5 Be assertive, *not* aggressive. Assertiveness simply means standing up for your rights. Aggression involves trespassing on the rights of others. Put forward your views clearly and firmly, but never indulge in personal attacks. Having made your concern or displeasure clear, work with the teacher to see what practical steps can be taken to resolve the problem.

6 Try seeing the situation from the teacher's position. Ask yourself what you would feel, think and do if you were in her shoes. This makes it more likely that you can negotiate an outcome that satisfies everyone.

7 Be willing to do as much listening as speaking. Don't be so eager to put over your views that you are deaf to what the teacher has to say.

Ask questions if you don't understand something, or request clarification for any comments which seem unreasonable. If you disagree with what has been said, say so, and politely explain why. Never fall into the trap of trying to flatter, appease or agree with teachers just to stay on good terms with them.

How do you talk to teachers?

Award a point for any statements with which you agree:

1 I have a quick temper.
2 I prefer to avoid anything unpleasant.
3 I do not suffer fools easily.
4 I often feel guilty, for no good reason, when talking to policemen.
5 I hate waiting in a queue.
6 I have difficulty talking to strangers at a party.
7 I usually complain about shoddy goods or poor service.
8 I am shyer than most people.
9 I always say what I think.
10 I am unsettled by changes in routine.

Total your score for odd- and even-numbered statements separately. If you scored highest on odd-numbered statements you respond with aggression when stressed. The higher your score, the more aggressive you are likely to become. This means you could try harder to stay cool in any discussions with your child's teachers.

If you scored highest on even-numbered statements you are too easily browbeaten. The higher this score, the harder it is for you to cope with a confrontation. Don't be afraid of asserting yourself where your child's future is concerned.

Equal scores for odd and even numbers mean that you become aggressive in some situations and anxious in others. Try to stay calm and stay assertive in all your encounters.

Anxiety over failure and achievement

School, with all the stresses and challenges which it imposes, makes a great many children feel very anxious. Sometimes such anxiety is fleeting and not especially handicapping – little more than apprehension before a test or feeling nervous when criticised by a teacher. But for many students, a great deal of the 15,000 hours spent at school is made miserable by chronic anxieties. And, contrary to popular belief, such anxiety is rather more likely to be suffered by higher-achievers than those doing less well in class. In fact stupidity is actually used by some children as a means of defending themselves against lack of success.

How failing reduces fears

While being branded a dunce may not do much for a child's self-image it can work wonders for anxiety. Once a pupil has been labelled a failure, teachers tend, not surprisingly, to expect little of them and make few demands on them. They are less likely to be asked questions or have their queries taken seriously. Mistakes and failures to understand their lessons are considered an inevitable consequence of their lack of ability.

As a result they are able to idle their time away at the back of the class. So long as they don't interrupt the teachers or distract other students, their presence may pass almost unnoticed through lesson after lesson. Failing children often form a distinct sub-culture within the school – groups of under-achievers who employ various defence mechanisms to protect themselves against the anxieties their lack of scholastic success might otherwise produce. The comments below, together with the defence mechanisms each suggests, are typical of those made by classroom drop-outs.

'Nobody could learn with such bad teachers.' (Mechanism: projection.)

'You don't need exam passes to make a lot of money.' (Mechanism: rationalisation.)

'I can get any job I want without doing well at school.' (Mechanism: denial of reality.)

'What matters most in life is luck, and I'm a lucky person.' (Mechanism: undoing.)

'When I don't like a lesson, I just bunk off.' (Mechanism: real-life avoidance.)

'I often daydream through lessons I find hard.' (Mechanism: fantasy avoidance.)

Reassuring one another that lessons are a waste of time, that studying is useless and exam passes pointless, these classroom failures drift through their school days armoured against anxiety – yet doomed to almost certain failure in adult life.

The eighteenth-century poet Thomas Gray caught their situation perfectly when, in *Ode on a Distant Prospect of Eton College*, he wrote:

> Alas, regardless of their doom
> The little victims play,
> No sense have they of ills to come,
> Nor care beyond today.

How anxiety brands children stupid

The decline into classroom failure is frequently due not to any lack of intelligence on a child's part, but to a tragic self-fulfilling prophecy of inadequacy, often triggered by that child's initially high levels of anxiety.

As I explained in Chapter Two, performance and anxiety are linked by an inverted U-shaped curve (see page 36). As arousal increases, so too does achievement, but only up to a certain point – the Peak Performance Stress Level (PPSL). Beyond the peak of the curve, however, increasing arousal leads to a catastrophic decline in one's ability to think clearly or act efficiently.

A child whose early days in school are marred by sufficient anxiety to take him well above this PPSL will *appear* less clever, capable or competent than less anxious fellow students. And it does not take long for teachers to arrive at a clear, and usually enduring, judgement about his or her intellectual ability.

Once branded bright or dull it takes a great deal of evidence to the contrary to change teachers' perceptions of a child. Even when presented with clear evidence that a child they regard as stupid is actually of normal, or even above average, intelligence, the initial assumptions tend to remain.

Instead of reassessing the child's ability in the light of the new facts, various 'explanations' will be offered. For instance, the teacher may believe that the child cheated, that his homework was done by parents, or that he arrived at the right answers through lucky guesswork. Teachers are not alone in falling into such traps. Research has shown that we all make fairly rapid judgements of one another, usually within the first few minutes of the initial meeting, and that, having made up our minds, we are very reluctant to change them.*

Regarding a child as not very clever subtly influences the way in which teachers respond. In a study of the influence of adults' assumptions on their response to children a twelve-year-old boy was given individual tuition by teachers who were told one of three things about the boy. Some were informed that he was extremely bright, others that he was a reasonably clever child and the remainder that he was unintelligent. Their teaching sessions with him were then video-taped.

It was found that when the pupil was regarded as highly intelligent the teacher's attitudes and, especially, their body language were significantly different from when they believed him to be either average or dull. They gave him more eye contact, stood closer to him, were more tolerant of mistakes and allowed more thinking time after asking a question.

So the child whose anxiety has branded him with a dull label is very likely to find himself treated differently from his or her fellow students. In this way a self-fulfilling prophecy of failure is created.

Need for achievement versus fear of failure

Children who do very well in class, get good marks in all their tests and excellent exam grades may pay an unacceptably high price for their attainment. These are children whose success is motivated by a *fear of failure* rather than a healthy *need for achievement*.

The 'need for achievement' child
Children with a strong need for achievement are not over concerned about making mistakes. They tackle novel tasks

*See *In and Out of Love*, David Lewis, Methuen, 1987.

with enthusiasm and confidence, even when not entirely sure what they should be doing. When they suffer setbacks or failures they learn from them and seldom make the same error twice. They enjoy new situations, fresh challenges and unfamiliar activities.

'Need for achievement' children are able to assess their chances of success realistically. While this does not prevent them from tackling difficult tasks, they are unwilling to waste their time on anything which is clearly beyond them.

The 'fear of failure' child

Children with a strong fear of failure, by contrast, tend to dislike anything unknown. They are cautious and conservative in their approach to novelty and prefer to stick to what they know and can do well. Failures or errors make them very upset. Instead of learning from their mistakes, they try hard to avoid that activity in the future. They like what they know, and what they know they can do well at. They set themselves easily achieved goals, and need to be constantly reassured of their attainments.

Surprisingly, 'fear of failure' children often embark on what are clearly near-impossible tasks, where their chances of success are virtually zero. This seemingly paradoxical behaviour is easily explained. When the task is impossible to accomplish, the child cannot be blamed for failing. Indeed, he or she is more likely to win praise for being so 'plucky' and 'having a go'.

Suppose an indifferent swimmer announces that he will swim the Channel for charity. Nobody expects him to accomplish this, but many will applaud his courage and determination. If, however, he set himself a more realistic target – such as six lengths of the local swimming pool – his failure would clearly be blamed on his lack of stamina and skill. Fear of failure can lead to considerable classroom success in secondary education, but it is an unwise strategy for two reasons.

Firstly, the price paid in emotional distress can be extremely high. Some 'fear of failure' children literally burn themselves out by their late teens. At this point they are unable to continue in education and drop out, with their resistance to anxiety destroyed. Their attitude is often cynical, bitter and apathetic.

Because they are constantly running scared, such children can suffer a wide range of physical ailments and be extremely moody, depressed and irritable – all signs of excessive stress. It was fear of failure which transformed Martin Brown, the six-year-old whose story I told in Chapter One, from a confident pre-schooler into a sad pupil.

The second problem is that strategies based on fear of failure may allow children to prosper in the structured learning of secondary education. Here, clear goals for attainment are set and children know exactly what is expected. But once they move into higher education the lack of structure, less tangible goals and the need to be self-motivated in their work make it far harder for them to assess their levels of achievement.

As a result they feel confused and unappreciated. They are also handicapped by their reluctance to take intellectual risks and tackle problems where there are no right or wrong answers. This legacy of a fear of failure is one of the main reasons why youngsters who obtained good exam grades and were highly thought of by their teachers while in school may fail miserably when they go to university.

If your child scored 5 or more points on the 'Meeting expectations' and 'Coping with anything new or unfamiliar' sections of the assessment it is possible he, or she, is motivated more by a fear of failing than a need for achievement. If this is the case, here are six ways to help.

1 Reward your child for successes, but never be too critical of failures. When mistakes are made handle them in a neutral manner. Encourage your child to examine the mistakes she has made carefully and objectively, instead of trying to forget all about them. Confronting failures is never pleasant, but it can prove highly instructive. We usually learn more from our blunders and initial errors than we do from a first-time flawless performance.

Studies by Dr Richard Teevan of the State University of Albany, New York, has shown the mother's role to be especially critical here. When she punishes failures but responds in a neutral manner to successes, a fear of failure is very likely to result.

The PIN approach helps you strengthen your child's motivation while, at the same time, correcting mistakes. PIN stands for Positive, Interesting, Negative, and that is the order your comments must take.

Always begin by looking for and commenting on all the Positive features in your child's efforts. Sometimes it may be rather hard to discover very much that is worthy of your praise, but with persistence you'll always find at least a couple of positive features.

Next consider anything Interesting about his or her work. That is, original features, a novel idea or a new way of expressing a familiar thought.

Only then, when you've exhausted all the positive and interesting aspects of your child's work, should you seek out those Negative aspects which demand constructive criticism.

Sadly, this is *not* the way most adults comment on a child's work. All too often they launch into criticisms right away, and only then – if the child is lucky – search for anything praiseworthy. As a result many children simply stop listening as soon as a grown-up starts talking. They know from bitter experience that the comments are most likely to be negative and hurtful. So they avoid the anxiety which this would produce by switching off. As a result helpful and worthwhile remarks are missed.

By praising before nit-picking you'll capture your child's attention and help him learn important lessons.

2 When praising be sure that your comments are sincere and not excessive. A child who receives lavish praise for trivial accomplishments either loses trust in the adult or else believes that success is easily gained.

3 Reward far more than you punish. Research by Dr Kaoru Yamamoto of Arizona State University suggests that the best balance is achieved when there are five rewards to every one punishment. If you are uncertain what balance you are maintaining, keep a record, over the next couple of weeks, of every reward and every punishment you offer. Rewards include praise, encouragement, congratulations – even a warm smile at the end of a task. Punishments mean not only

a smack or being sent to bed, but telling your child off, being negatively critical, sarcastic, dismissive or indifferent; even frowning in disapproval counts as a punishing response.

If you find the balance is less than five rewards for every punishment, your child may be despairing of ever satisfying you. He or she is certainly much less likely to be approaching life in the risk-taking, curiosity-satisfying manner essential for developing intellectual skills and avoiding harmful anxiety.

4 Let your child's motto in life be, 'If a job's worth doing, it's worth doing badly.' That may seem terrible advice, but the fact is that only somebody willing to make mistakes, and then learn from them, is able to progress. Every learning task attempted, from speaking a language to playing sports, will be done badly before it can be done expertly.

Children, with a high fear of failure, though their aversion to novel or unfamiliar tasks, frequently deny themselves the opportunities needed to learn new skills and acquire further knowledge.

5 Never call your child 'stupid', 'idle', 'lazy' or any of the host of other denigrating words so often bandied about in home and classroom. I call such comments GIGO remarks, from the expression in computing: 'Garbage In, Garbage Out.'

This is a warning to computer programmers that if they feed rubbish into the machine, rubbish is all they can expect to emerge at the other end. The same applies, with even greater force, to the developing brain of a child.

What parents and teachers really mean, of course, is that a piece of work was done without sufficient thought or care. But by presenting comments about the quality of a piece of work as a judgement on the child they can do serious harm to a youngster's self-image. Children who are told repeatedly that they are 'stupid', 'clumsy', 'careless' or 'bad' internalise these negative descriptions until they see themselves in the same terms. A circular argument than develops with the child explaining away a poor standard or work, or unacceptable conduct, by claiming that it reflects his true potential or personality. 'I am naughty in class, because I am a naughty boy,' says James, aged nine.

Adults too fall into the same trap. 'John is a stupid child,' a teacher may tell you. How does he know? 'Because John does bad work in class.' Why does he do bad work in class? 'Because he's a stupid boy.'

That the argument is pointless and purposeless seldom seems to occur to those advancing it to 'explain' a child's behaviour. Furthermore, it prevents any more sensible search for the true reasons for a child's failure from being conducted. These mistakes and misbehaviour often stem from preventable anxieties. Once these have been identified and resolved, the 'stupid' child suddenly makes great intellectual strides and the 'naughty' youngster becomes a model student.

6 The best way of encouraging children with a fear of failure to become more adventurous is to devise tasks where some risk of failing is involved. These need to be very carefully selected, since if they are too hard to accomplish your child may grow so anxious that performance is undermined. Then her lack of success merely confirms her desire not to take such risks in the future. On the other hand, if the goal is so easy to accomplish that no genuine challenge is involved, your child will gain little satisfaction from its attainment. These activities need not be intellectually demanding to enhance intellectual performance.

I shall never forget the look of triumph on the face of eleven-year-old Danny as he successfully navigated a canoe down a rapidly flowing river. The boy, a chronically anxious child with a pronounced fear of failure, had believed himself quite incapable of managing the course. But patient and skilled coaching took him to the point where he was willing, under a certain amount of firm but friendly pressure, to have a go. This success was a major factor in transforming his fear of failing into a strong, positive need for achievement.

If you feel your child might be helped by this strategy, be sure to follow these guidelines.

* Be patient. Build slowly towards a tough ultimate goal.
* Be persistent. Encourage your child to go at a pace just slightly faster than he feels comfortable with. Not so fast that he starts to panic, or so slowly that the goals achieved are seen as trivial.

- Be careful. You need to be 90 per cent certain that your child can accomplish the ultimate goal before allowing an attempt to be made.

One way of safeguarding him against ignominious failure is to set a goal which is more than he believes is attainable, but less than you judge he is capable of achieving.

In the river race, Danny's coach was fairly sure that he could complete the whole, hair-raising course through white water. But he was absolutely certain that he could reach a point halfway down. So he set that as Danny's goal, and assured him that he would achieve it. 'When you get there,' he added, 'keep on going if you want.' Danny's delight in his final success was greatly enhanced by the fact that he had accomplished more than his coach had, apparently, considered possible.

Remember that you cannot hand your child success on a plate. Do that and you are offering a valueless gift. The only success worth having is success that has been earned.

Using fantasy training

You can use Mind Movies, at the end of a relaxation session, to help a fearful child tackle activities which are currently either avoided, or where anxiety is impairing performance. After guiding her through the mind-quieting image – of the desert island or whichever other scene she favours – switch to the activity that is causing difficulty.

Help your child imagine the situation so vividly that, as well as seeing it in his mind's eye, he also experiences it through the senses of hearing, touch and, where appropriate, taste. If he starts getting upset during the Mind Movie, immediately switch to the relaxing scene. Then, when he is calm again, return to the anxiety-arousing scene. By repeating this fantasy training on several occasions you can greatly improve his ability to cope with the situation in real life.

Helping with homework

The time will come when you child starts bringing back homework, and this can be a cause of considerable anxiety.

For Mary and her eight-year-old daughter Felicity, homework was often hell. The little girl became anxious and frustrated when she couldn't understand a subject, and made her distress known either by furious rages or by weeping with misery. 'I'll never understand it,' she would yell in despair.

Mary badly wanted to help, but felt defeated by subjects she had never learned in school. If you face the same problem, there are some practical ways to help.

Start by recognising that homework matters. It is not simply an irritating invasion of your child's free time. Educational researchers have shown that pupils who work successfully at home do better in class and achieve higher marks in exams.

To do his homework properly, your child must have a quiet place to study, preferably a room to himself without the distractions of a TV or a family chatter. If this is impossible, try organising a rota system with parents whose children have a similar problem. One night a group of children do their homework at your house. For the occasion the TV is kept off, and other members of the family stay out of the room. For the remainder of the week, your child goes to somebody's else's house.

Set aside a specific time for the homework. This should be after your child has had a chance to relax, but before supper. The brain works much less efficiently after a heavy meal. It is not a good idea to watch TV for more than thirty minutes prior to homework, since viewing reduces alertness and impairs concentration. In one American study, children were connected to equipment which automatically switched off the programme when their mental and physical alertness dropped beyond a certain level.

Although the children were eager to watch the show, a cartoon, the longest any could remain sufficiently alert to keep the set switched on was thirty seconds. After that they became so inattentive that the machine was shut down. Some psychologists now believe that the growing inability of US students to pay attention in class is due to excessive TV-watching. This is not a result of the actual programmes being viewed, but of the way in which the image is built up on the television screen. As you probably know, this is achieved by a rapidly moving dot which is used to build up the picture. It has been found that watching this type of image produces electrical rhythms in the brain which are associated with a more relaxed mental state.

By comparison, a short period of brisk exercise, such as fast walking or a vigorous game, makes body and brain more alert and thus able to function with greater efficiency.

If your child has just started doing homework, and is not very well organised, it may be helpful to check what has to be done as soon as he gets home from school. That way, if reference books are needed or things like paper, pens etc. have to be purchased, you'll still have time to visit library and shops before they close.

When your child gets stuck and asks for help it is important to provide this in the right way. Clearly, just giving her the answer is pointless. Not only does this prevent her from learning the subject, but it also causes teachers to assume that she knows more than is the case. When facts have to be looked up from books, show her how to use references rather than finding the information for her yourself. Provide practice by asking questions similar to those in the homework assignment, and then helping her dig out the answers. The ability to locate facts and figures in a wide range of standard references, such as dictionaries and encyclopedias, is a skill every child should master as early as possible.

If you are demonstrating the best way to solve a problem, be certain you understand exactly how to do so before you start. As I shall explain in the next chapter, believing that an adult cannot understand their work either causes many children to become very anxious.

Make certain that you are using the same problem-solving procedures your child has been given at school. Even if your method is efficient, it can still confuse a child who has been taught an entirely different way of tackling such problems. Study your child's textbook carefully and practise answering set problems privately before attempting to demonstrate them to your child.

Never provide answers for the homework questions.

Instead, invent similar problems that can be used to illustrate the best way of finding answers.

While helping, remain calm and patient, even when your child makes what seems to be a stupid mistake or careless error. Such practical assistance will help to transform what is often an anxiety-arousing ordeal into a positive learning experience. You can often prevent homework dramas by asking the following questions as soon as your child gets home.

- What subjects have you got to study for homework tonight? Have you got the school books you need? When your child has just started doing homework, and may still be slightly confused about what is entailed, it is often safer to go through these books with them in order to make certain.
- Are any additional reference books necessary? Again, with a younger child, glance through the tasks to be done.
- Is any special stationery needed?
- Are any craft materials, card, glue, paints etc. wanted?

Of all the subjects your child learns at school, and you may be asked to help with at home, the one which causes the greatest dread in most households is arithmetic. It is also the one which creates the highest levels of anxiety in children. Many fail dismally when it comes to maths, yet such failures are mainly caused not by a lack of ability but by overwhelming anxiety. In the next chapter I shall explain what you can do to help.

Twelve
Helping To Banish Maths Anxiety

There can be few more anxiety-arousing subjects on the school timetable than maths. The majority of children fear and loathe it, while even educated men and women often have difficulty in solving the most basic number problems.

A study by Bridget Sewell of Reading University concluded that 30 per cent of adults suffer from arithmophobia, an intense and irrational terror of numbers. Where simple sums are concerned, the least success is achieved by the sixteen-to-twenty-four age group, with those aged forty-five to sixty-four forming the next largest group of poor problem solvers.

Her survey revealed that nearly half the UK adult population cannot read a railway time table, one in three are incapable of dividing sixty-five by five, while a further third are unable to do simple multiplication and subtraction.

Thirty per cent of those interviewed could not calculate a 10 per cent tip on a restaurant bill, or understand that if a store was offering a 25 per cent discount customers must still pay 75 per cent of the original price. Only two in ten appreciated that if inflation fell from 15 per cent to 5 per cent, prices would continue to rise. Interviewers reported that many of those questioned were made very anxious by being asked to do sums, and half of those approached refused even to attempt the questions.

If your child is currently having difficulties with arithmetic, it is likely that he or she also dreads the subject and becomes confused, anxious and uncertain when confronted by figures. It may also be that your own memories of arithmetic lessons are far from happy and that you too lack confidence when it comes to sums.

Bridget Sewell's report concluded by saying that many people are put off arithmetic at an early age. The comments made to one of my researchers by a 27-year-old shopkeeper undoubtedly express the experience of many. 'As a kid I used to be in tears because I couldn't understand how half times a quarter equals – whatever it equals. It took hours and hours of teachers showing me and I still couldn't grasp it at all – I felt a failure. You just lose confidence really, and it can affect you through other things as well. If it's not caught early you never get it right.'

In her book *Overcoming Math Anxiety* Shiela Tobias remarks that the first thing people remember about failing at maths is that

> ... it felt like sudden death ... failure was sudden and very frightening. An idea or a new operation was not just difficult, it was impossible! And instead of asking questions or taking the lesson slowly, assuming that in a month or so they would be able to digest it, people remember a feeling, as certain as it was sudden, that they would *never* go any further in mathematics.

If you share this experience and these sentiments, it is likely that when your child complains about how impossible maths is to understand, and how much he dislikes it, you respond sympathetically.

'I could never do sums either,' a mother says comfortingly as her son stares incomprehensibly at his maths homework.

'I shouldn't worry too much about your poor exam results,' comforts the father who also dislikes working with figures. 'Most people do badly in arithmetic.'

How curious that, where numbers are concerned, poor comprehension and low attainment are regarded as somehow inevitable and acceptable, while a similar lack of understanding and achievement when working with words would bring down the wrath of protesting parents.

A ten-year-old who announces that she cannot solve

maths problems because of difficulties with numbers earns sympathy and understanding in many homes. But if the same child were to comment, casually 'I can't read very well, I'm no good at understanding letters,' her bland admission would almost certainly be met with shock and alarm. Illiteracy is shameful, innumeracy socially respectable.

When it comes to negative attitudes and excessive anxiety affecting classroom performance, therefore, the classroom skill at greatest risk is maths.

Maths avoidance

If given any sort of number problems, many children immediately switch on one of the defence mechanisms which I described earlier. They may refuse even to attempt the challenge (avoidance) with the brisk, dismissive comment that, 'I can't do sums.' Or, when compelled to make an attempt, they might adopt a modified form of avoidance by dashing through the calculations as fast and as unthinkingly as possible.

They have little idea of what they are doing or why, don't know when or why an answer is right, or how or where the error lies if it's wrong. This is a worldwide problem. A Russian child explained his method of arriving at an answer by saying, 'I add, subtract, multiply and then divide until I get the answer that is in the back of the book.'

Children may rationalise their failures by insisting that, 'Nobody can do sums.' Or they may deny the reality of the subject's importance: 'Nobody needs to do sums.'

Parents also resort to similar strategies: they avoid thinking about their child's failings, claim that they've done perfectly well in life without knowing any maths, or project the student's failure on to the teacher's inadequacy.

The latter strategy, combined with justified concern over poor progress, leads many parents to spend money on additional coaching. While this can be helpful for some children, in other cases it simply undermines the child's limited number skills even further. The anxious, poorly motivated youngster with a poor self-image where maths is concerned is merely made more fearful and less motivated by out-of-school coaching. His self-esteem drops even further, as he comes to see himself as a maths dunce.

So what can you do at home to help your child be less frightened by figures?

It would take an entire book to do full justice to this complex problem, and for readers interested in taking the matter a great deal further I can recommend Sheila Tobias's *Overcoming Math Anxiety.** Although written for the American market, this book contains a wealth of helpful advice. There are, however, some practical ways of reducing your child's arithmetic anxieties and enhancing his number skills which can be more briefly described.†

1: Avoid self-defeating talk

I have already described some of the unhelpful comments which parents make when sympathising with their child's maths difficulties. While kindly intended, any remarks which reinforce your child's negative image of himself as being incapable of ever understanding arithmetic do him a great disservice in the long term.

A large part of the problem stems from a widely held belief that there is such a thing as a non-mathematical mind. As Sheila Tobias points out, it is curious that nobody ever talks about children having a 'non-historical' or a 'non-geographical' mind.

There are, of course, a very small number of children who certainly possess 'mathematical' minds. Saul Kripke, for instance, was still a young child when he worked out, for himself, the equation $(a - b)(a + b) = a^2 - b^2$, simply by playing with numbers and observing that $(5 - 2)$ multiplied by $(5 + 2)$ was equal to the square of the larger number minus the square of the smaller $(25 - 4) = 21$.

Similarly, William James Sidis, the American prodigy whose IQ was estimated at being 100 points higher than Einstein's, solved complex equations in front of senior

---

*Published in America by Houghton Mifflin in 1978. A good UK bookshop will get it for you.

† A cassette training programme based on this chapter is available. See Appendix.

students while still so small that he had to stand on a stool to reach the blackboard.

The fact that a tiny minority of youngsters have especially well-developed maths ability does not, however, mean that the majority of children have non-mathematical minds. Given persistence, encouragement, self-confidence and freedom from crippling maths anxiety, almost every child is capable of enjoying considerable maths success.

So the next time your child comes to you complaining that the subject is difficult, worrying, incomprehensible or hateful, do not go along with that statement. Instead, provide practical help in getting to the bottom of the confusions or misunderstandings.

2: Check your own knowledge

The topics covered in your child's maths classes have probably changed a great deal since you were taught. Subjects like topology and statistics, now a routine part of secondary education, may not have even been mentioned during your schooldays, while procedures have also changed.

This means that even if you were fairly good at maths at school, you could still find yourself floundering when trying to help your child. If your knowledge and confidence is limited, well-intentioned but fumbling attempts to assist with homework may only leave your child more anxious than before. 'If Mum and Dad can't do it,' she reasons, 'what hope for me!'

So before making any attempt to help, read through the school texts and classroom notes carefully. Work through examples in the textbook, and be sure that you understand each link in the chain of reasoning.

If you are not particularly good at maths you may be reluctant to assist through fear of making matters worse. In fact, parents who have to work hard to solve sums themselves, but who persist until they have gained a thorough understanding of the subject, frequently make far more successful teachers than those skilled at maths. When an activity comes easily to us, it is harder to remain patient with the blunders of a beginner. As the Russian writer Alexander

Solzhenitsyn has perceptively remarked, 'A warm man never knows how a cold man feels.'

Those who have had to struggle to gain understanding are better able to appreciate the confusions and uncertainties of a child striving to acquire the same knowledge, so never be deterred from helping your child because of worries about your own poor performance at school. Provided that you do your homework, and really understand what you are going to teach before embarking on a lesson, your child can only benefit.

A few schools are now offering places in class to parents interested in knowing more about their children's lessons. Grown-ups are able to sit alongside their child and be taught by the same teachers. In other schools teachers are sometimes prepared to arrange 'remedial' maths classes, after school, for groups of interested parents. This is a possibility well worth raising with your child's school, if your are really interested in understanding his or her maths homework.

3: Common difficulties you can resolve

Fairly major mistakes and confusions in arithmetic at secondary level often result from quite minor errors or misunderstandings at a much earlier stage in the child's studies. Maybe she missed, or never really grasped, a fundamental fact taught at primary school. The gap in her knowledge went undetected for years but, like a weakness in the foundation of a skyscraper, the more knowledge she built on that insecure footing the more serious the crash when it came. Here are three common sources of error which you do not have to be any kind of maths genius to eliminate.

Errors of procedure
All problems contain three essential components, known technically as Givens, Operations and Goals.* In a maths problem the Givens are the numbers involved, together with the student's knowledge about the way those numbers can

---

*For a full discussion of these terms see my book *You Can Teach Your Child Intelligence*, Souvenir Press, 1981.

be manipulated – e.g. multiplied or divided. Such knowledge is usually assumed to be stored in the student's brain, although in some exams certain complicated formulae will be given.

The Operations are the things you do to the Givens, and the Goal is the answer required. In the example '3 × 6 = ?' the Givens are 3, 6 and the 'x' sign, indicating which operation to perform. The Operation consists of multiplying the numbers to arrive at the Goal, which is to replace the '?' with a number.

From secondary level onwards, these three components are seldom so obvious in maths problems. However, they are still there, and if your child fails to solve a problem it is because he or she has not understood one or more of them correctly. You can help identify errors in procedure by setting your child sums of the type he finds hard and then getting him to work through them with you.

If this diagnostic session is going to be helpful, instead of merely making your child even more anxious – almost all arithmophobes hate being watched while they work – it is essential not to be impatient or critical. Use the listening procedures described in Chapter Seven. Keep your tone friendly and encouraging at all times. It often helps to start by setting sums you know your child can solve, thus enhancing assurance and motivation.

I am not pretending that building confidence between a previously critical adult and a maths-anxious child is easy. It takes time and persistence before he or she is prepared to admit to not understanding something.

Making a tape recording as your child talks her way through finding the answer to a problem can be extremely helpful. It allows you to notice any negative self-talk and identify sources of difficulty for future reference.

As your child talks herself through the answer-seeking process, speak as little as possible yourself, and never criticise a mistake – however silly it seems to you.

Do not attempt to correct a mistake either. By doing so you could prevent an even more serious misunderstanding from coming to light. The time to explain where her reasoning was faulty is after you have identified all the mistakes, not before.

Once you are satisfied that you know what errors in reasoning, or false assumptions, underlie her wrong answers invent problems – or find them in your child's textbooks – which provide the practice needed to overcome that particular weakness.

You may find, for example, that your child still uses what is called a 'counting up' method to find the answer to simple sums, such as 5 plus 8, where one of the numbers is less than 10. Sometimes when he is 'counting up' you can see his lips or fingers moving slightly to keep a check on the addition. All children use this method when first learning to do maths, but it is important that the process becomes automatic as soon as possible.

If you were asked to add 4 and 8 you would, hopefully (!), immediately 'know' the answer was 12 without having to count. The danger of using a 'counting up' procedure is that errors can easily creep in. If your child is older than eight and has still not automated the process of adding two numbers, one of which is less than 10, you should provide practice by playing number games involving this skill.

Errors caused by zero

A second common source of difficulty for many children is the concept of zero. Before reading further, jot down your own idea about what 0 means in maths. Mathematics teacher Knowles Dougherty comments: 'If you ask an obedient child in the first grade, "What is zero?", the child will call out loudly and with certainty, "Zero is nothing." By third grade, he had better have memorised that "Zero is a place-holder." And by fifth grade, if he believes that zero is a number that can be added, subtracted, multiplied and divided by, he is in for trouble.'

Here's how seven-year-old Mark explained a mistake in his sums, based on an incorrect understanding of zero: 'You can't take 1 away from nought because nought means nothing, and you can't take something away from nothing. So the answer is nought.'

The idea that by writing a 0 you are saying that there is nothing there may sound like nothing more than common sense. I have even heard teachers fall into the same error. But to write nought into a calculation is to say something more subtle than simply stating that 'nothing' is present. Zero is a number just like 1, 2, 3, 4, 5. Technically, it defines the 'number of elements in the empty set'.

It tells us that no members of a particular group are being counted. The group might be a collection of books, or toys, or apples, or children. In the number 160, the 0 tells us there are no '1s' present in the '1s' column. In the 102 it indicates that no 10s are present in the 10s column. In 1022, it says that no 100s are present in the 100s column.

This is not, however, the same as saying that nothing is there at all. To say that a field contains 'zero sheep' is simply to make the point that *no sheep are present*; it tells us nothing about other things which might be there, such as cows, trees or birds. In other words, the field can be full up with anything and everything in the world, except sheep.

You may feel this is so obvious that it hardly needs stating, yet errors based on a failure to understand the concept of zero commonly arise from this simple misunderstanding. Until resolved, this will continue to plague a child in all aspects of arithmetic, from addition and subtraction to multiplication and division. If a child persists in the belief that zero and nothing are one and the same, then even fairly basic and straightforward calculations become impossible to carry out correctly.

Should you discover that your own child has a similar confusion, it is essential to correct this error before any progress in arithmetic can be made. Fortunately it can usually be banished quite easily by a teaching session lasting just a few minutes.

An easy cure for zero errors
Start by collecting some objects such as toy bricks, apples, oranges and so on. Place them on the table, then sit down with your child. As in any teaching session, it is important to keep the atmosphere friendly. Here's how Mark's mother, Jean, resolved his confusion. She began by giving him two simple subtraction problems, one involving a zero answer: $4 - 4 = ?$. The second required the subtraction of zero: $4 - 0 = ?$

After Jean had shown Mark the sums, the following conversation took place:

Jean: 'Can you solve these two problems for me?'

Mark: 'Yes, that's easy . . . the answer is nothing for both of them.'

Jean: 'Well, suppose I were to give you four oranges . . . then take them all away . . .'

Jean placed four oranges on the table in front of him and then removed them again. By using real objects at the start you make it easier to illustrate the points being made. The next step is to move from real objects to words, by writing the names of the objects. Finally, you move from words to numbers and represent the objects with integers.

Jean: 'How many do you have now?'

Mark: 'I haven't any at all.'

Jean: 'That's right. But even if I did that, you couldn't say you had nothing, could you?'

Mark: 'I don't understand what you mean.'

Jean: 'You'd have your clothes, and your toys, your books and pencils. All you could say was that you didn't have any oranges. [Taking a sheet of paper she writes a nought followed by the word 'oranges'.] 'That's just another way of telling somebody how many oranges you had after I took them all away. Now suppose I gave you four books. Write down how many you have.'

This time she writes the word 'books' on the paper and gives it to Mark.

Jean: 'Just write the number in front of the word 'books'.

Mark confidently writes 4.

Jean: 'Good, suppose I took the four books away from you. Can you write down the number that tells me how many books you'd have left?'

She writes the word 'books' again and hands the paper to her son.

Mark: 'I wouldn't have any books left, so I'd write down a nought.'

Jean: 'That's right. Well done. This time I want you to pretend that I've given you another four books [she writes the number 4 on the paper] but I don't take any away. [She writes the number 0 under the 4 and puts in a minus sign.] Can you do 4 take away 0 and write down how many books you would have left?'

Mark: 'That's easy, I'd still have four books.'

Jean: 'That's very good. You are quite right. But when I gave you the problem of 4 minus 0 a few moments ago, you wrote down 0, didn't you. Now you understand why that was wrong.'

Mark: 'Yes, but before you explained I thought that 4 minus 0 must be nothing.'

Jean gives Mark six further problems to consolidate his understanding. If there are any mistakes, she repeats her explanation until his confusion over zero is resolved. She continues to give him zero problems during the next few weeks to keep the idea fresh in his mind.

The next stage is to eliminate any difficulties which arise when zero forms part of a number, as in 120 or 102. Explain that a 0 in the 1s column just means that there are no 1s in that number, e.g. 120. A 0 in the 10s column means that there are no 10s, e.g. 102. A 0 in the 100s column means that there are no 100s, e.g. 1022, and so on. In less than five minutes this procedure allows you to banish confusions over the concept of zero from your child's mind.

Errors over words

Misunderstandings can arise when a child fails to understand the meaning of terms employed. For instance, a little earlier in the chapter I used, without explanation, the term 'integer'. The sense in which it was given should have told even those unfamiliar with the word that it means a whole number. Specifically, an integer is any whole number, whether positive or negative (e.g. 1, 2, 3 or – 1, -2, -3). But a child who did not understand what 'integer' meant might well fail to solve a problem which, had he understood the term, could have been solved with ease.

Another common confusion surrounds the word 'multiply'. Children learn, early on, to expect that multiplying something means to make it bigger. Yet when they start working with fractions of less than one, they discover that multiplying them produces a smaller, not a larger, fraction, e.g. $\frac{1}{2} \times \frac{1}{2} = \frac{1}{4}$. Because this appears to contradict what they have previously been told, many become perplexed and anxious. They struggle to produce larger fractions and so become hopelessly confused.

Again, the term 'of' generally implies division to find a portion of some quantity, for instance a half of 10 means $^{10}\!/_2 = 5$. But where fractions are concerned, 'of' tells you to multiply, not divide. A $\frac{1}{2}$ of $\frac{1}{10}$ solved by multiplication and not division.

Another common source of error, identified by Sheila Tobias, is in the word 'cancel' used in connection with fractions. Children are instructed to 'cancel numerators and denominators' but, as she points out, 'Nothing is being "cancelled" in the sense of being removed for all time.' Incidentally, the words 'numerators' and 'denominators' can themselves be troublesome. Some children fail to carry out the calculations correctly because they confuse the number above the line in the fraction, the numerator, with the denominator, the number below the line.

Negative numbers, such as −5 or −1, can also present grave difficulties to children who are convinced that a − sign always means subtraction. They have to taught the new meaning of the minus sign before they can even begin to understand such problems as $-1 \times -1 = ?$

4: Start early

The sooner you can sort out any confusions in your child's understanding of maths, the better.

Mitchell Lazarus suggests that there is a 'latency stage' in learning maths, during which a child's misunderstandings can pass unnoticed, not only by his teachers but by the child himself. For a while he continues to do quite well by adopting a 'cookbook' approach to problem-solving. He slavishly follows a set formula to reach the answer, without any idea how or why the end result is arrived at.

'Because his grades have been satisfactory,' says Lazarus, 'his problem may not be apparent to anyone, including himself. But when his grades finally drop, as they must, even his teachers are unlikely to realise that his problem is not something new, but has been in the making for years.'

So check your child's work regularly, looking not just at the answers but also at the methods used to arrive at them.

5: Make arithmetic meaningful

The sad thing about failures in maths is that people who regard themselves as virtually innumerate can still manipulate numbers with speed and confidence in some areas of their lives. Darts-players, for instance, can calculate scores accurately and at high speed, while many teenagers who run a mile from a maths book make models which require very precise measurements. Children who are duffers in the arithmetic class can weigh and measure ingredients in cookery without difficulty. A twelve-year-old boy in one of my study groups was hopeless when dealing with numbers on a page, but could work out complicated sums when giving change in the charity shop where he helped out on Saturday morning.

The more that you can make number problems practical and relevant to your child's life, the more confident and motivated he or she will be in solving them. As a result anxiety is greatly reduced, while speed and accuracy are enhanced. As I explained in an earlier book,* only around 23 per cent of children have the kind of brains which work best when dealing with abstract problems, the sort children are most often given in class. The remaining 77 per cent are disadvantaged not because they are dull or dumb but simply by the way in which certain lessons are taught. By teaching your child maths in the way best suited to his personal learning style, you will find that the skills are mastered far more easily and willingly.

6: Encourage guessing

A sign in one maths classroom read, 'No guessing allowed'. This is poor advice. While wild guesses are unhelpful, educated ones are part of every professional mathematician's

---

* *Mind Skills*, Souvenir Press, 1987.

toolbox. As Joseph Warren has commented, 'Mathematicians use intuition, conjecture and guesswork all the time except when they are in the classroom.'

By learning how to make an educated guess at the likely answer, your child can better judge whether her answer is correct or wildly out. This is especially important when calculators are being used, because it is easy to become confused about the magnitude of the correct answer.

When I was at school, slide-rules rather than silicon chips were the main tool for long calculations. They were slower and less convenient, but had two major advantages over calculators. Firstly, you had to know where to put the decimal point; the slide-rule did not do it for you. This made errors of magnitude caused by an incorrect placing of the point less likely.

Secondly, answers were only calculated to 2 or 3 places of decimals, for instance 3.142 for the value of pi. Calculators can give you pi to as many as 9 places of decimals – 3.141592654 – which looks far more impressive and accurate than 3.14 but for practical purposes in school maths is meaningless. In other words, the child is beguiled by rows of numbers into thinking that his answer must be correct because it looks so impressive.

A good guess helps put the answer into perspective. For instance, if you multiply 16 × 5,000 what sort of answer can be expected? The child who guesses at an answer between 50,000 (5,000 × 10) and 100,000 (5,000 × 20) is going to be more certain that his calculated answer of 80,000 is correct. A child who has not made such an educated guess and is presented with the number 80000.0000 on his calculator screen may have no idea whether it should be 8,000, 80,000 or 800,000.

Finally, do not be too hard on a child who has to struggle to make sense of maths. Many of the early mathematicians, whose contribution helped shape modern mathematical thinking, were unable to cope with concepts that today's children are expected to cope with as a matter of course. The early Greeks, for example, found the idea of zero so confusing that they could only resolve the dilemma by banishing nought from their numbering system. Considering what superb mathematicians the ancient Greeks were, it should come as no surprise to learn that, two thousand years later, many children still find difficulty in solving problems which include a zero.

Parents whose children are having trouble understanding the idea that −1 × −1 = +1 might feel less concerned over such a failure if they knew that the great German mathematician and philosopher Leibnitz, whose discovery of calculus in the seventeenth century helped put men on the moon in the twentieth century, was also unable to accept the idea of negative numbers.

The history of man's slow and painful understanding of mathematics frequently repeats itself as children struggle to come to terms with ideas about numbers which once baffled the world's greatest thinkers. Just as the knowledge of those early scholars was forged from their initial misunderstandings and mistakes, so can your own child's knowledge develop from current difficulties and confusions to clear understanding and worthwhile attainment.

Thirteen
Helping Achieve Exam Success

Anxiety, rather than a lack of either intelligence or ability, is probably the main reason why so many children do so poorly when taking exams. Physical and mental tensions impair memory, reduce confidence and act as barriers to efficient problem-solving. But it is not enough simply to teach your child how to relax when taking exams. To ensure examination success he or she must also know how to make the best use of the available time, both while revising for and sitting the exam. The recall of information must be rapid and accurate despite the pressure. Having one's mind go blank when faced with exam questions, only to remember every fact and figure perfectly once the examination has ended, is an all-too-common experience.

Only once these intellectual skills have been mastered, and confidence built up, will the relaxation procedures for reducing the symptoms of physical anxiety, and the Mind Movies for preventing negative thoughts, prove fully effective.

Planning for success

Revising for an exam is rather like training to run a marathon. The sooner your child gets into shape, the better her chances of completing the course successfully. If possible, revision should begin at least six weeks before the first exam, so that the studying can be done in short, regular sessions spread over many days rather than – as so often happens – being crammed into a few, frantic days.

Although your child will, naturally, need to spend more time on especially difficult subjects, it is important to avoid the mistake of thinking that because a particular subject is easy there is no need to revise it. This sort of misplaced confidence has made many students do badly in the very exams where everybody – themselves included – expected an excellent result. It is equally unwise for your child to neglect subjects he finds especially difficult in the belief that, since he is bound to fail anyway, revising it would only be a waste of time. By working intensively on a poorly understood topic students often find that they can make sense of it after all.

To help with the considerable self-discipline needed for successful revision, your child should keep a record of studying progress by preparing a timetable on a large sheet of paper which can be pinned up in the room where he does his revision.

Create the planner as follows. The number of days remaining until the first examination are written down the left-hand side of the sheet and the subjects, or topics, being revised along the top. Vertical and horizontal lines are then drawn to create a rectangle for every subject against each of the revision days.

Now your child must decide how many hours each day can be spent revising. This will obviously depend on the amount of other work which has to be done at the same time. I suggest that he only works for six days a week, and sets aside the seventh for rest and enjoyment. He might decide, for instance, that he can set aside two hours for revision on every weekday and four hours on Saturday. This means that he will be revising for a total of fourteen hours each week. Each revision session should last not more than twenty minutes, with a ten-minute break between each study period. By working for short periods memory is enhanced, concentration improved and motivation more easily sustained.

Allocating time in this way means that your child can complete two revision periods per hour. Next, calculate how many study periods can be completed per week. This is done by simply doubling the number of hours set aside for revision. If, for example, fourteen hours a week seems a realistic amount of time to set aside for revision, twenty-eight study periods are possible.

Next, discuss with your child the number of study periods to allocate to each subject. A straightforward way of doing this is to divide the number of study periods available by the total of subjects being revised. If your child has twenty-eight periods available and is revising four subjects, then seven study periods could, in theory, be allocated for each. It is usually advisable, however, to set aside more time for complex subjects.

For instance, your child might decide to devote ten sessions to arithmetic, eight to chemistry, six to history and four to geography. The first allocation of time should only be seen as provisional, and can be modified as revision progresses. Your child might find that some subjects are harder to revise than expected, while others are easier, so reallocate study periods accordingly. Bear in mind, however, that all subjects being examined must be revised.

As your child completes each study period he should tick, or block in, the appropriate box on his timetable. This enables him to see at a glance the progress being made. By colour-coding different subjects he can also check that sufficient revision time is being given to each.

Here's how it might work in practice. Suppose your daughter starts a two-hour study period at 5 o'clock in the evening. Her first revision session will finish at 5.20. She must be disciplined over the allocation of time – this is excellent practice for the actual examination – and never finish either much before or too long after the end of a session. A kitchen timer or the alarm watch can be set to provide a warning when time is up. It must also be emphasised that during this period she must concentrate fully on her revision.

If she intends to study another subject during the next period, she should use the break to tidy away her notes and references for the first one and prepare the material needed for the next period. That done, she should leave her desk and spend the remaining time relaxing. Walking around the room or doing stretching exercises during breaks helps reduce any bodily tension created by studying. This is specially helpful towards the end of the revision sessions.

If there's time she can listen to some light music or glance at a mentally undemanding book or magazine. The great thing is not to reflect on what has just been learned. By diverting the mind from the topic studies, memory of it will be improved and there is less risk that facts from one subject will get muddled up with information about the next.

Once again, self-discipline is central to success. When the rest period is over, she should return immediately to her revision. After working for another twenty minutes she can take her second, ten-minute, break. As before, old notes should be tidied away, those needed for the third study period prepared, and mind and body generally relaxed. The ten minutes remaining at the end of the final revision session should be used for putting away study materials.

If your child is studying for longer periods, say four or six hours, revision time should be broken into blocks lasting two hours each, with a twenty-minute rest period between each block. A sample timetable, for a four-hour session starting at 4 o'clock in the afternoon, is shown below. Although it may seem that your child will be wasting rather a lot of time by taking so many breaks, she will actually learn far more successfully because her brain is being allowed to work with greater efficiency.

Managing examination time

A student once remarked that the shortest five minutes in the world are the last five minutes at the end of an exam. In order to avoid not finishing, or having to rush the last answer attempted, it is essential that your child learns how to allocate time during the examination with care and self-discipline.

An attempt must be made to answer all the questions asked. Some students believe that first-class answers to two out of four questions will compensate for unanswered questions and are a better way of approaching exams than

Time allocation for a four-hour revision session		
		Start 4.00 p.m.
Period One	20 minutes	4.20 p.m.
Break	10 minutes	4.30 p.m.
Period Two	20 minutes	4.50 p.m.
Break	10 minutes	5.00 p.m.
Period Three	20 minutes	5.20 p.m.
Break	10 minutes	5.30 p.m.
Period Four	20 minutes	5.50 p.m.
Break	20 minutes	6.10 p.m.
Period Five	20 minutes	6.30 p.m.
Break	10 minutes	6.40 p.m.
Period Six	20 minutes	7.00 p.m.
Break	10 minutes	7.10 p.m.
Period Seven	20 minutes	7.30 p.m.
Break	10 minutes	7.40 p.m.
Period Eight	20 minutes	8.00 p.m.

Complete revision, tidy away study materials.

giving average answers to all four. In fact you could answer half the questions very well indeed, yet still fail. A simple calculation makes clear why this is so.

Suppose your child has to write four essays of equal length. This probably means that a possible 25 marks can be earned from each. If only two are attempted the maximum mark possible is 50 and, since it is virtually impossible to obtain this for any essay answer, the actual marks will almost certainly be less.

Suppose that 20 are awarded for each essay – still a good mark – giving your child a total of 40 per cent. This represents a low pass mark in some examinations but a failing grade in others. But if all four essays have been written and awarded, let us suppose, 15 marks each, your child would have achieved 60 per cent, or a very good pass.

It is vital, therefore, that your child decides how much time she will allocate to the various questions and then sticks to that plan during the exam. Past papers, experience during mock examinations and guidance from teachers will give your child this information.

Make sure she attends the exam equipped with an easy-to-read watch, and encourage her to keep a close eye on the time. Even when she can answer one question far more fully than the others, she should never be tempted to devote more time to it than her plan allows. Suggest that she divides up the time available as follows:

Start by reading the questions carefully and deciding which can be answered. Prepare her for the fact that, on first reading, all may seem confusing and beyond her. Reassure her that this is a perfectly normal reaction, and should not lead to panic. By using the anxiety-management procedures described in earlier chapters, and the memory-enhancement skills I shall outline in a moment, your child should find it fairly easy to remain calm and recall the required information to mind.

The way in which she allocates time to questions will vary according to the nature of the paper. For example, let's suppose that there are four essay questions of equal complexity to be answered in two hours. Here's how a time management plan for that examination might look:

Reading the questions carefully – two minutes. This time is crucial to success. Many candidates fail because they give excellent answers to a question which was never asked.

Next prepare an 'ideogram' from which to answer the first question chosen. I shall describe this powerful technique for enhancing memory on p. 182. It allows your child to recall the necessary facts and figures with ease and produce a well-structured answer that includes all the relevant information. Time allocated, three minutes.

Then write the essay – allocate twenty minutes for this.

Finally check the essay – five minutes. This final step must not be neglected because careless errors can easily creep into the answer and will cost marks unless detected and corrected.

Thirty minutes have now passed.

Time should be allocated for subsequent essays in exactly the same way. Your child should attempt to finish the final essay with five minutes to spare, in order to be able to reread all her answers briefly.

Time is your child's most precious possession during an exam. Encourage her to use every second wisely and fewer.

Studying for success

Have you ever found an answer by forgetting the question? You want to remember a name or a quotation, and although it's on the tip of your tongue you just can't bring it to mind. Then, some time later, the fact suddenly surfaces. When this happens you have experienced your brain's unique knowledge network in action. This contains every item of information you ever learned. What happens is this:

Once instructed to find a piece of information, your brain diligently searches through the memory files for it. Since every fact you know is linked to all the other facts, the mind is able to trace a pathway from one idea to the next. Sometimes facts are very close together in a particular file. For instance, if you are asked, 'What colour is a canary?' You should immediately be able to answer, 'Yellow'. This is because the idea of a canary and the idea that it is yellow are intimately associated on the knowledge network. It is like having one fact in the first folder of a filing cabinet and the second fact in the next folder along.

Suppose, however, that you were asked, 'Is a canary an animal?' Now you take longer to answer because the two items of knowledge are not located in adjoining folders of the same file but in different cabinets entirely. Questions like this were posed by the American researchers Collins and Quillan, who carefully measured the time taken for people to answer. They found that the more closely items were associated, the briefer the search time needed.

To make sure that your child is capable of fast, error-free recall during exams, he must organise what is learned into concisely structured knowledge networks, where the links between key facts are short and direct. This is how to do it.

You will need several dozen plain cards, a large storage box and some coloured pens. The method can be used for any subject where there are considerable numbers of facts to be learned. It is suitable for revising English literature, history, geography, biology, some aspects of chemistry and physics (but not formulae) and religious instruction. It is not helpful for maths or foreign languages.

(The last two subjects can only be learned by constant rehearsal and practice, but the more relevant the problems posed, the easier storing and retrieving the knowledge will be. For instance, rather than learning a list of nouns in a foreign language, make the subject come to life by speaking, reading and listening to the words. Where formulae are concerned, never try committing them to memory until you understand them. Once they make sense, retention is far easier and recall more likely to be accurate.)

Step One
Select a subject to be revised and decide which are the major topics to be covered. Past papers, advice from teachers, classroom notes and chapter headings in books will help your child make this selection.

Step Two
With the major topics identified, your child must now search out key information related to each one. These essential facts are written on cards, one card to each fact.

Extracting and recording the information has to be done with great care since, once extracted, it becomes your child's sole revision source. Notes must be brief and very much to the point. Practise yourself by digging for key facts and figures from one of your child's texts before trying to explain the procedure. Abbreviations, drawings or sketches can be used to compress facts on to a card, which should never contain more than about forty words. If a fact is too long and complicated to be reduced in this way, it must be broken down into shorter items of information. Write words in *red*, use *green* for drawings, while numbers, symbols, figures, formulae etc. should be noted in *blue*. These colours will help to boost your child's memory.

Step Three

With the cards prepared, those relating to a single topic – let's say the Battle of Hastings – should be selected. Your child can start with any card, which is placed face up on the table. Now he selects a second card containing a fact which relates in some logical way to the information contained on the first card. A third card is selected in the same way and laid down on the table. Other cards are added to create a circle, with the last card placed next to the first one. There should be between fifteen and twenty-five cards in the circle. Any fewer, and too little information will be memorised at a time; many more, and the task of recall will become needlessly hard. Experiment with the number of cards, however, since some children prefer to work with more cards and some with fewer.

In the history example, a card containing notes about where the Battle of Hastings took place might be followed by cards detailing who led the Norman and English armies. By creating a circle of key fact cards, your child transforms lists of facts into a knowledge network which has neither a beginning nor an end. This means that recalling any fact makes it possible, by mentally travelling around the circle, to bring to mind any other.

Step Four

Your child's next task is to transfer those facts from the knowledge network into memory. By preparing the cards he has already organised and stored away a considerable amount of information, so the task of learning those facts will be far easier.

Starting anywhere he wishes on the circle, and moving in either a clockwise or anti-clockwise direction, your child now reads the information contained on each of the cards in turn. As he does so, encourage him to form mental images of the information – to see the facts not just as words on a card but as vivid pictures in the mind.

He proceeds around the circle, reading each fact in turn, until he is back at the starting-point. This process is repeated two or three times. Now the facts are read again, but as each is noted that card must be turned over. When all the cards are face down it is time for your child to try and recall the information in that knowledge network.

He flips over any card he likes, reads the fact it contains and attempts to remember the facts on the cards either above or below it in the circle. He should remain relaxed while doing so, allowing the knowledge to bubble up from the depths of his mind. Should he become stuck, and this is very likely during early trips around the network, he simply turns the card over and reads out the fact.

When he has recalled a fact, your child turns the card over to check the accuracy of his recall. After all the facts have either been remembered, or cards turned over and the elusive information read, the whole procedure is repeated.

Your child should use different starting points on the network and vary the direction of travel around the circle, sometime moving clockwise and sometimes anti-clockwise, though having begun moving round in a certain direction, he must continue in that direction for the remainder of the recall session. After just a few trips around the network, he will be able to remember all the facts it contains quickly and accurately. Furthermore, recalling any one fact will enable him to bring to mind every other item of information.

Step Five
Your child may also find it helpful to record himself reading out the facts, and then play the tape back during odd moments like travelling to school. By storing facts in his visual, sound and muscle memories – the brain remembers which hand, wrist and arm movements were used when writing something down – your child significantly enhances his retention and recall.

The more actively he works with the material to be revised, the easier – and more interesting – studying becomes. So encourage him constantly to ask himself these questions about the information:

'What are the key facts or issues?'
'How did things happen?'
'Where, when and why did they happen?'
'Who was present?'
Once he can answer such basic questions without reference

to the notes, his understanding of the topic is sound, and confidence over being examined in it should significantly improve.

After completing a revision session all the cards relating to a particular topic should be filed away in clearly labelled envelopes and carefully stored. Depending on the complexity of a subject, and the depth to which your child has to learn it, there could be from two to twenty sets of cards for any particular subject.

Envelopes containing topics within a subject area are best kept together in a separate box. For instance, History revision cards should be kept in one box, Geography cards in another. Inside each box one might find, in the case of the History box, for example, envelopes containing cards about major battles, kings and queens, princes and priests, political reformers and social changes.

If your child doesn't understand a particular topic, he should not attempt to try and memorise it. Instead, help him pinpoint the cause of his misunderstanding or confusion. Has he failed to grasp a vital fact at an earlier stage in studying and is it this gap in his knowledge which makes it so hard for him to understand later information?

Suggest he checks over the notes and references, and asks his teachers for guidance and clarification. He should never feel shy or embarrassed about doing this, since the time to say you don't understand is while revising, not when sitting the exam.

Step Six

Creating knowledge networks not only makes revision far easier and less anxiety-arousing; it also provides a valuable tool for constructing answers during the exam itself.

Having read the question very carefully, your child should take a sheet of scrap paper and quickly jot down anything he can recall about the subject. Tell him not to get anxious if his mind goes blank, but to remain calm and focus his attention on the topic in a relaxed manner. He should picture himself setting out the network cards relating to that topic during revision.

Because of the structured way he has organised that

knowledge, recalling a single fact from the relevant network will allow him to remember all the rest of the information it contained. As each fact is recalled, it should be quickly scribbled down on the paper.

When sufficient information has been recovered, these notes can become a blueprint from which to create a well-organised answer. Your child finds a suitable fact with which to begin the answer, draws a circle around it and numbers it 1. Now he finds a second fact which follows logically from the first, and numbers it 2. He continues in this way until all the facts needed for the answer have been identified and numbered. The results is an *ideogram*, which provides the foundations on which an answer is built.

By spending a few minutes on this preparatory work he ensures that no key facts are missed from his essay and that his ideas are clearly presented. Effective presentation, which provides evidence that the student has thought about the subject instead of simply regurgitating facts, adds significantly to marks.

This procedure can improve your child's chances of success in another way as well. If candidates are allowed, or required, to hand in rough notes with the answer papers your child should always include his ideograms, having first crossed them out clearly to indicate that they are merely working notes and not part of his final answer. The advantage is that, if he included facts in his ideogram which, for some reason, he forgot to include in his answer, he might still gain credit for the knowledge. If, however, there are any mistakes in the ideogram, but not in the actual answer, no marks are going to be lost. So your child cannot lose anything and might gain a vital additional mark.

Managing exam nerves

Use the relaxation procedures taught earlier in the book to combat exam anxiety. After your child has unwound physically and spent some time picturing himself or herself in safe, comfortable surroundings, the Mind Movie should switch to the examination room. Younger children may need to be guided through the procedures; older ones often prefer to do it for themselves. Your child should picture herself on the day of the exam – getting up and dressing, eating breakfast and then travelling to where the exam is being held. She should imagine herself, as vividly as possible, entering the exam room, taking her seat and preparing to start.

As in all Mind Movies, images should be accompanied by sounds, sensations of touch, smell and taste. She hears the scraping of chairs as candidates sit down, the rustle of paper as questions are read, the relentless ticking of the clock.

If any of this makes your child anxious, she should immediately switch back to the relaxing scene and unwind. When mentally and physically relaxed again, she can return to the imaginary exam room.

During these training sessions she must picture herself staying calm and confident in the examination room. Feeling slight apprehension, but avoiding excessive anxiety. She can also practise experiencing, and rapidly bringing under control, anxiety created by any particularly stressful moments during the exam, such as reading through the questions or realising that time is almost up. The calming effect of gently massaging the forehead or bringing to mind Floppy Bear should also be employed. Mind Movies should be practised well before the first exam. By working through them in fantasy, she will find that real-life exams are far less frightening.

She should be sure to relax physically the night before her exam, and immediately on waking up the following morning. If possible, another brief relaxation session immediately before going into the exam room is beneficial. She should find a quiet spot and spend a few moments sitting quietly, allowing her muscles to unwind and calming her mind with a soothing image.

When sitting in the exam room, she should relax as much as possible, noticing any needless bodily tensions and easing them away by imagining the anxiety flowing out of her body, through her fingertips, and vanishing into the room. A quick method for fairly unobtrusive relaxation is as follows:

1 Clench and relax the fingers.
2 Shrug and release the shoulders.

3 Roll the head around the shoulders three times in each direction.
4 Frown and press the tip of the tongue to the roof of the mouth.
5 Flatten the stomach and stretch the legs.
6 Take a deep breath, exhale slowly and as the air escapes imagine oneself growing more and more relaxed.

These powerful procedures will prevent anxiety from ruining your child's chances during exams. They should also boost confidence, enhance self-esteem and help sustain motivation.

Now let's consider what your child should be doing during the final run-up to the big day.

Countdown to the big day

With two weeks left
Check he is on schedule with his revision. Have all the subjects being examined been allocated time? Remember that he must revise actively, by asking himself questions, making notes and using visual imagery to strengthen recall. Past exam papers can be used to test knowledge and practise answering questions in the time allowed.

Be careful of his health. It is important that he takes plenty of exercise in the fresh air and eats sensibly, including fruit and vegetables in his diet. He should avoid drinking too much tea or coffee while revising, since this can impair memory during the exam.

Relaxation and Mind Movies should be used regularly to develop a positive, anxiety-free attitude towards the challenge.

With two days left
He should concentrate on his first two exams, going through all the relevant fact cards at least once.

Is he sleeping well? A relaxation session when he gets home should help him get a good night's rest.

With one day left

Prepare a checklist of all the things needed in the exam room. Does he have a spare pen? Are the batteries in his calculator fresh? A little advanced planning builds confidence and helps him approach the challenge with far greater assurance.

With only one day to go there is no reason, if he has revised methodically, why he shouldn't take the day off, forget his studies and enjoy himself.

Before going to bed, make sure that everything required for the big day is at hand.

On the big day

- Make certain that your child leaves home with plenty of time to spare, so that if anything should go wrong, such as a train running late or a bus failing to arrive, she won't panic.
- Encourage her to eat a good breakfast, since this helps reduce anxiety. Include an egg, fish or meat as well as bread or cereals, because protein will help her body digest food more efficiently and ensure that energy levels remain high throughout the day. She must not drink more than one cup of coffee or tea, as caffeine is a potent stimulus which greatly increases the risk of exam nerves.
- Last-minute revision is best avoided. Instead, she should just read calmly through summary cards to jog her memory.
- Sucking a glucose sweet or eating a few raisins before going into the exam room gives the blood-glucose level a boost and helps make the mind more alert.

During the exam

She must remember to read every question carefully. If unable to answer a short question she should move straight to the next, going back at the end if there is time. Research shows that pondering a tough question not only wastes time but also increases anxiety.

If completely baffled by a multiple-choice question tell your child to take a guess. Studies show that this is the best strategy when the answer really eludes her.

She should never worry about how others are doing, but concentrate solely on her own paper.

After the exam

Discussions about the question paper are very tempting but best avoided. If your child's answers differ from others she could become depressed and anxious, perhaps for no good reason. The best advice is to forget an exam the moment it is finished and concentrate on the next one.

By mastering these easily learned skills, and using relaxation combined with Mind Movies to control anxiety, your child should find that examinations are no longer a terrifying barrier to success but a challenge which, with care and effort, they will meet successfully.

Fourteen
Helping Your Phobic Child

How your child's phobia develops

One of the most famous children in the history of psychology is an eleven-month-old orphan known only as Little Albert. More than half a century ago he was the unknowing subject of a research project which, while it will disturb many parents, proved a milestone in our understanding of how phobias can develop.

In 1920 an American psychologist named John Broadus Watson used Little Albert in a classic demonstration of how children – and adults – become phobic. When he was first given a tame white rat to play with, the little boy showed only delight. After observing his behaviour for a while, and noting the fearless way in which he approached and handled the rat, Watson stood close to the child with a hammer and a sheet of metal. Every time Little Albert reached out to stroke the rat, Watson banged the metal loudly, startling and scaring the infant.

After a while, the fright caused by the ear-splitting banging was triggered by the sight of the rat. Soon Little Albert reacted with fear whenever the rat was produced. Even the sight of it made him cry and crawl anxiously away. Little Albert had been conditioned to feel an irrational terror of white rats. He was phobic about them. (You will be relieved to know that Watson later removed the fear as effectively as he had created it, using the same approach that I shall be describing in this chapter.)

If your child has a phobia, you may well recall some incident which, like Little Albert, caused him to be afraid. Perhaps he met a large, unfriendly dog who responded to his eager approach by growling or snarling. Later, the fear this dog had aroused made him try to avoid even a small, friendly puppy. Perhaps you unintentionally made him fearful by your own behaviour – showing fear when, for instance, there was a thunderstorm, your child grazed his knee or a spider fell into the bath.

As we have seen already, anxiety is a perfectly natural and normal response on which our survival often depends. Its purpose is to help us avoid, or be very careful with, anything in life which is hazardous or harmful. The greater the threat, the higher the levels of anxiety aroused and the stronger our desire for escape or avoidance.

While we are born with a knowledge of 'how' to fear written into our genes, there is no similar blueprint telling us 'what' we ought to fear. This is the result of learning. It depends on what we hear, see, taste, touch and experience; on what our parents, teacher, brothers or sisters, relatives and friends say and do. From these exchanges with the world at large we come to fix a 'fear this' and 'avoid that' label on certain things.

It is also true, however, that we are born with greater vulnerability to some things than to others. For instance, when other researchers tried to make children phobic about objects such as coloured bricks or hairbrushes, using Watson's technique, they were far less successful than he had been with Little Albert. It seems we have an inborn tendency to become more fearful, more readily, of things which move than of inanimate objects. This makes perfect evolutionary sense, of course, since moving things are far more likely to pose a threat to survival than stationary ones.

Freud distinguished between 'common phobias' – which he saw as an exaggerated fear of all those things which most people to some extent detest or fear, such as being alone, death, illness, snakes, heights or blood – and 'specific phobias', which he described as 'the fear of special circumstances that inspire no fear in the normal man'.

A child who is terrified of climbing to the top of a tall building, therefore, is only showing a normal, sensible fear in an exaggerated form. But a child who is too petrified of a caged bird to go into his granny's flat because she has a pet budgie would have a slightly different kind of phobia. However, whether common or specific, these fears can be tackled in exactly the same way.

Now let's see how a frightening incident can turn into a phobia. It is only common sense to realise that people are more likely to repeat some action when rewarded than if punished for doing so.

This everyday observation has been analysed in great detail over the past fifty years and given the name The Law of Effect by psychologists. The Law simply states that when someone does something which has a positive result, the chances are that they will want to repeat that action. If your young son washes the dirty dishes without being asked, and you immediately show your pleasure and approval, he'll be more willing to wash up again. But if you either take no notice of his helpful act or criticise him for not getting the plates clean enough, he'll think twice before lending a hand again.

Although this sounds so obvious that it hardly needs saying, the link between being rewarded and repeating an action is a good deal more complicated than most people realise. Suppose, for instance, you say nothing at the time, but give him a rise in pocket money at the end of the week. Will this:

a: be less effective than a word of thanks immediately after the washing-up is done?
b: be more effective than immediate praise?
c: have no effect on his future actions?

Or what if you sometimes praise your child for washing up, but on other occasions ignore him? Will this make it:

a: more likely that he'll wash up again?
b: less likely?
c: have no effect on his behaviour?

In both cases the answer is a. All the available research shows that what matters is not, within reason, the size of the reward but how quickly it is offered. Furthermore, irregular, unpredictable rewards have a more powerful effect on behaviour than regular, predictable ones.

You can see the proof of this any time you watch people playing fruit machines in pubs and clubs. These machines are designed to make payments randomly but instantly. No player can ever tell how many times the handle must be pulled in order to receive a pay-off, but they know that when they do strike lucky, their reward will be immediate. The tumblers click up a winning sequence and the gambler is greeted by the joyous sound of coins cascading into the delivery tray.

Where do those winnings go? More often straight back into the machine than into the gambler's pocket. Psychology sides with the fruit-machine owners, rather than the punters. The Law of Effect has conditioned players to keep on pulling the lever and watching the wheels spin.

This discussion of fruit machines may seem to have taken us a very long way from your phobic child. In fact, exactly the same principles apply.

Anxiety, as we have seen, is painful. Avoidance, as I have also mentioned, is a defence mechanism which either rapidly reduces the distressing mental and physical symptoms of anxiety or prevents them from arising. So avoidance is rewarding. Furthermore, the relief it brings is usually immediate.

Here's how it might work in real life. Your child wants to stay up and watch TV; you feel she should go to bed. There's a family fight. The row makes you anxious. You agree that she need not go to bed for another half hour. You have been rewarded, by the removal of anxiety, for giving in. Your child has been rewarded, for making a fuss, by being allowed to watch more TV. Both rewards were immediate.

The Law of Effect now tells us that, when the same situation arises in future – and you can bet that it will – it is more likely than before that your child will kick up a rumpus and you'll let her have her way.

A phobia can develop and be sustained in the same way. Here's what could happen.

Your child gets afraid in some situation – for example, when a fierce but chained dog barks at him. The next time he is either in the same situation, or thinking about getting into it, anxiety arises. Your child avoids it in some way. The anxiety subsides. Your child is rewarded. The next time the same situation occurs, avoidance is more likely than confrontation. Every avoidance makes further avoidance more probable, and the intensity of the anxiety experienced greater.

Now imagine that you must decide whether to compel your child to face up to that fearful challenge or not. Sometimes you insist and force him to go ahead despite his distress. At other times you feel so upset and sorry for him that you give in and allow the avoidance to take place.

Even if you only give in one time out of ten, this will still prove rewarding enough to maintain the pattern of anxiety and avoidance. This doesn't mean that you must immediately force your child to do something which, because a phobia has developed, causes intense fear. This would be not only cruel but completely unproductive. What it does show is that, once you have started on the training programme for removing fears that I am now going to describe, you must persist with it. Any backsliding will not only increase the risk of undoing all the good that has been done, but could leave your child even more fearful than before.

A practical plan for banishing phobias

Before implementing this plan your child must have learned how to relax her body, and have practised mind movies with you to the point where she can imagine scenes quite vividly.

Once these essential skills have been mastered, here is how to proceed. Although – as I explained in Chapter One – both children and adults can suffer from a wide range of phobias, research has shown that the vast majority respond well to a training programme based on the same general principles. Because your child's phobic difficulties were originally caused by avoidance, the only way to eliminate these difficulties is by helping him confront and cope with situations that currently arouse anxiety.

In this plan you will be encouraging your child to do things which make him feel some anxiety, not terrified but slightly apprehensive. The method can be likened to the correct way of training for a marathon. The wrong approach would be to run as far as physically possible on the first day and stagger home utterly exhausted. The next morning, with every limb aching, you would probably decide that running was beyond you and vow never to exercise again.

The sensible strategy, of course, is to build stamina progressively so that you avoid ever becoming too exhausted or distressed. For an unfit person, the first few training sessions may involve nothing more strenuous than brisk walking. When this can be accomplished without difficulty, short bursts of jogging are added. Gradually, over a period of days and weeks, the amount of time spent running rather than walking is increased. But at no time is the body placed under excessive stress through over-strenuous workouts. In this way physical health is slowly but surely improved. There may, of course, be occasions when we are tempted to run too far or too fast and, the following day, feel stiff and cramped. Instead of discouraging us, this should simply serve as a warning to revise the training schedule and make slightly slower but steadier progress.

When helping your child overcome his or her phobia you will be adopting the same step-by-step approach.

Set a goal

The starting point is to establish, through discussion with your child, the ultimate goal to be accomplished. It is important to define this goal clearly and precisely, otherwise one cannot create an effective plan for getting there.

For a child with claustrophobia an ultimate goal might be to travel up several floors in a small lift. For a youngster with a dog phobia, the ultimate goal might be cuddling a friendly dog. When the parents of nine-year-old Sally, the spider phobic, talked over their daughter's fears with her she said that her aim would be to catch a large spider in a glass and put it outside. She believed that this was quite impossible, and even felt anxious having to talk about it.

On a sheet of paper write TARGETS in large letters, and then note your child's ultimate goal at the top.

Make a list of sub-goals

Your next step is to identify a series of sub-goals which will take your child, slowly but surely, towards that ultimate goal. These sub-goals can be compared to stepping-stones across a wide river. The success of your child's self-help programme lies in placing these stepping-stones at just the right distance from one another: too close and his progress may be so slow that you'll all get bored and discouraged; too far apart, however, and there's a risk of his falling into the river. Your child may become so anxious when attempting to complete a sub-goal that he'll give the plan up as impossible.

By talking quietly and sympathetically to your child you should be able to discover some activity related to the phobia which causes only slight apprehension. Write this down at the bottom of the TARGETS sheet. Above this place a second activity which your child feels would be harder than the first. Add a third sub-goal, an activity which your child says would be even more difficult for him to tackle – perhaps so hard that, at the moment, it seems impossible to achieve. There should be at least four sub-goals between your starting point and the ultimate goal.

Draw boxes around each sub-goal and then join these oblongs up with vertical lines so that they form the steps of a ladder which takes your child – in slow, easy stages – from starting point to ultimate goal. Do not be surprised or concerned if your first attempt at creating the programme proves unsatisfactory in some way. It may be that the steps have been placed too far apart, which means that your child will feel too much anxiety while attempting to progress up the ladder. Equally, some of the sub-goals may prove too close together, slowing progress. But, always remember, it is very important that your child feels some slight anxiety when first attempting each situation. It is only by experiencing, and controlling, the mental and physical symptoms of anxiety that the phobia can be overcome.

Rate anxiety

Assess the appropriate level of anxiety by asking your child to rate his or her feelings in each situation on a scale of 1 to 5, where 1 means there is no anxiety at all, and 5 that he starts to panic. Select a situation which scores around 3.

Sally's plan in action

Here's what Sally's plan for overcoming her spider phobia looked like. Her overall goal was to be able to catch a spider in a glass and remove it from the house.

The first sub-goal on her list was sitting in a room for fifteen minutes with a small toy spider placed on a table six feet away from her. As she sat in the chair, she went through the relaxation procedures her mother had taught her, noticing any needless tensions in her body, face, arms or legs and making them go loose and floppy. The relaxation countered any anxiety she was experiencing. Although nervous when she first sat down, Sally rated her anxiety at 4 on the scale, by the end of fifteen minutes it had declined to 2.

Her second sub-goal was to sit slightly closer to the spider, again relaxing while doing so. Sally rated her initial anxiety at 3 and her level of arousal at the end of the session was 1, indicating that she was not anxious at all.

For the third sub-goal she sat at the table with the toy spider only inches away from her. This led to an initial rating of 4, and a final rating of 3. Because of this she repeated the third sub-goal on two further occasions. Between real-life practice sessions, her mother took her through fantasy training using the Mind Movie technique.

With her daughter completely relaxed, she asked her to switch from the soothing mental image to picture herself seated at the table with the toy spider before her. Sally was told that if this made her particularly anxious she should raise a finger. On the first session she did this after only a few seconds of entering the scene. At this point her mother immediately stopped guiding her through the spider imagery and returned her to the beach. On the second session, Sally allowed her mother to talk about the spider for several minutes before indicating that she was starting to feel unpleasantly anxious. As before, the image was immediately 'turned off' and her mother instructed her to see herself back on the warm, sunny beach.

Sub-goal four involved touching the toy spider, while at sub-goal six she picked it up. Although Sally had been worried about touching the toy spider, and felt that picking up even a plastic replica would be horrible, in the event she was able to do both these easily, rating her anxiety at 3 for each.

Next Sally repeated the process with small, live spiders, gradually sitting closer and closer to them while they remained securely trapped in a jam-jar. On every session, which lasted fifteen minutes, she focused on feeling mentally and physically relaxed in the presence of the spider. After five weeks of regular practice every day, Sally was able to carry the jam-jar into the garden and set the spider free.

A slightly larger spider was then obtained by her parents, and the process repeated. Fourteen weeks after she started working with the plan, Sally achieved her ultimate goal. She was able to go into the bathroom and, using a tumbler and a sheet of paper, remove a spider from the bath.

She felt apprehensive about this but, thanks to the progressive way in which her anxiety had been brought under control, there were no real problems.

Your support is essential

Sally's parents were very supportive throughout this training. Although insisting that she practise every day – the closer together the sessions, the more quickly and easily progress can be made – they rewarded her on every occasion with praise and recognition of her efforts. This is absolutely essential to the success of the plan. Your child must feel that he or she is really accomplishing something worth while. If you are ever dismissive of the gains made, progress will be severely limited.

One twelve-year-old I was treating for a severe cat phobia was making excellent progress until his father – an army officer – returned from an overseas posting. When his son started to tell him, excitedly, how much easier it was for him to approach cats, the man sneered: 'I don't know what you're so pleased about. You should be ashamed of yourself for being frightened of cats in the first place.' As a result he gave up even trying to get rid of his fears, which five years later were still making life miserable.

In addition to praise, Sally's mother also gave her daughter more tangible rewards. After each successful session, the completed sub-goal was ticked off with a bright red fibre-pen. The TARGETS sheet was also pinned up on the door of the refrigerator so that her regular progress would be watched by the whole family. For every two ticks, Sally was awarded a token in the form of a gold star which was stuck on to the sheet. These stars could be exchanged for extra treats, more TV at the weekend or a small present. Remember that the more swiftly behaviour is rewarded, the faster it becomes established.

Use Mind Movies

Fantasy training using Mind Movies is very helpful, even when real-life practice is also possible. But it becomes of major importance when, because of the nature of the fear, practising in real life is either impracticable or impossible, such as with an interview or examination phobia.

You can prepare your child for handling the anxiety-arousing situation in real life by directing Mind Movies during which your child becomes only slightly apprehensive. It is important that some slight anxiety is experienced in order for your child to learn how to bring these feelings back under control. But if anxiety rises too high, she'll simply refuse to continue with the Movie.

Provide some means, such as the raised finger used by Sally, by which your child can indicate when anxiety is rising too fast, and then be sure instantly to switch off that arousing scene and return to mentally relaxing imagery.

During Mind Movies you can also help your child develop positive images which help him cope with the anxiety. Fearless Tiger proves a good friend to many younger children, who can imagine him at their side as they approach the feared situation. Linking Fearless Tiger to feelings of confidence during other training sessions, as described in an earlier chapter, will also help to boost your child's self-assurance.

Older children can contribute their own ideas for helpful images. When I asked an eleven-year-old what might make it easier for him to cope with his fear of dogs, he replied that imagining himself shooting past them on his new skateboard reduced his anxiety. So, in his imagination, I guided him on several trips down the street past a house where there was a large, unfriendly German shepherd dog. At first he was allowed to picture himself speeding past the house on his board. But gradually he slowed down until he was able to stop outside the house and watch the dog through the gate.

The confidence developed during fantasy training made it far easier for him to repeat the same actions in real life.

Mock situations

With thought, preparation and ingenuity it is often possible to introduce elements of real-life practice into most training programmes. A teenager who finds interviews a major challenge, for example, could be helped by practice at mock interviews where friends and relatives acted the role of interviewer. A fifteen-year-old with a phobia about speaking in public was helped by her parents, using a mixture of the procedures I have described. As her school's head girl she was expected to make a short speech to the assembled pupils and parents at the end of the school's open day. This terrified her so much that she even considered refusing to accept the honour of being made head of school. After learning to relax, she created a programme with 'making a confident presentation at the end of term' as her ultimate goal on the TARGETS sheet. Sub-goals consisted of making presentations to smaller groups. Clearly it was impossible to practise the final goal, since this would be a one-off event. However, she was able to stage-manage many of the sub-goals. Friends and relatives provided a small, sympathetic audience for short speeches.

At first these took place at home, then in a local hall which her parents hired for an hour to let her practise talking aloud in a much larger building. Her head teacher also allowed her to rehearse in the school assembly hall on a number of occasions. By having friends sit in different parts of the hall, she was able to practise delivering her speech loudly enough to be heard by all the audience. This helped boost her confidence. At the same time she went through regular fantasy sessions, in which she imagined herself making the speech in a clear, calm and confident manner. On the big day, although naturally slightly anxious (3 on the rating scale) she delivered her speech without hesitation and received loud, and well deserved, applause.

A sixteen-year-old boy with a phobia about flying was helped by visiting the airport, watching aircraft take off and land, and being allowed to relax inside a mock-up aircraft. Many airlines have these engineless fuselages which are used for training flight staff. If approached tactfully, and the flying phobia explained to them, airlines are often prepared to allow short visits to these training mock-ups. Being able to sit inside a replica fuselage and then, in a relaxed state, imagine the take-off, flight and landing makes it far easier to handle the real flight.

Help yourself as well

If you have a phobia yourself, why not use exactly the same procedures for getting rid of it? There are many good reasons for doing so. First of all, it is probably quite a nuisance at times, if only because it often makes you feel a bit silly. Secondly, as I explained at the start of the book, children can develop phobias after watching the way their parents react to various situations. By banishing a phobia from your life you'll be able to safeguard your child.

Finally, working through the programme will enable you to gain valuable practice before seeking to help banish your child's phobia.

Summary of the programme

Start by teaching relaxation. Show your child how to unwind the body and mind. Guide him or her through the pleasant imagery until these soothing scenes can be switched on at will. Use Fearless Tiger and Happy Hound, or similar images, to enhance confidence and happiness.

Create a list of fears, starting with a situation your child can handle with only a slight amount of anxiety, and work slowly but surely up to the ultimate target. Don't worry if your child insists that this is too terrifying to cope with under any circumstances. He will be able to do it by progressing up the ladder.

Finally, keep in mind these six important rules for making this phobia-fighting plan a success.

1 Be imaginative when helping your child create sub-goals and don't be afraid to ask other people – strangers as well as relatives and friends – to help you if necessary. You'll be surprised at how willing they are to co-operate.

2 Be prepared to rewrite your child's TARGETS list as the training progresses. If too much anxiety is being experienced, *add* additional activities. If your child can cope without any anxiety, *skip* a sub-goal.

3 Practise regularly. Short, daily sessions are far more effective than longer but less regular training periods.

4 Tick your child's TARGETS chart as soon as a sub-goal has been accomplished. Award some token, such as a star stuck on to the sheet, to reward accomplishments. Be very supportive. Have an especially nice reward for when the ultimate goal is finally attained, but never punish or be critical of your child for failing to achieve a sub-goal. All this means is that the stepping stones are too far apart. Find an intermediate sub-goal which can be accomplished.

5 There will be times when your child seems to suffer setbacks. A task which was tackled easily on one day will present problems the next. This is perfectly usual and does *not* mean that he or she will fail in the end. Be understanding but firm. Do not allow your child to avoid the activity. If it is being rated as too anxiety-arousing, return to the next sub-goal down on the list. If your child continues to practise regularly these obstacles will soon be overcome.

6 Fantasy training is very helpful even when the activity is also being tackled in real life. With younger children you may need to talk them through the Mind Movies. Older children will learn to direct their own, vivid mental images.

By following this easily implemented plan you should find little difficulty in freeing your child of a life-restricting phobia. And once banished it will never return.

Fifteen
Helping With Social Anxiety

One of the most common causes of social anxiety is bullying. This can start as early as nursery school or play groups. In a detailed study of nursery-school children, Professor Hubert Montagner of the University of Besançon has identified several different types of children by their position in the group's pecking order.

At the top are what he terms *dominant leaders*, youngsters who are able to organise games, dream up new activities and lead others without resorting to any sort of violence. Other children attempt to exert authority by throwing their weight around; Montagner calls these *dominant aggressives*. It is these children who, bossy and quarrelsome in the nursery, are most likely to grow up into bullies. As I commented in my own study of play group infants,* 'They grab, push and elbow their way through nursery life. They are seldom imitated, and only rarely start a game which others want to follow. Their aggression is often spontaneous and directed not against some child who has upset them but towards an innocent third party.'

Most often their victims come from a group of children described as *dominated frightened*. These children are like accidents looking for somewhere to happen. They tend to be overly submissive infants who make frequent attempts to

*The Secret Language of Your Child, Souvenir Press, 19??

appease or placate others. The pattern seen in nursery schools persists into primary and secondary education.

While bullies are usually larger, stronger and less academically successful than their companions, their victims tend to be quiet, diffident, over anxious and submissive. Since hitting back can, under many circumstances, lead to an escalation of violence, the best approach for your child to adopt is one of utter indifference. Although this takes time to learn, and demands a high degree of self-confidence and independence on the part of the child, it is the only tactic guaranteed to stop the bully in his tracks.

Bullies need helping too

The unhappiness of a bully's victim is often so heart-rending that an adult's first response is to give the bully a taste of his own medicine. This was Susan's immediate reaction when she discovered that her seven-year-old son Jamie had been mercilessly bullied by an older and bigger boy. 'I wanted to hurt him as badly as he'd hurt Jamie,' she confessed. 'Then I realised by doing that I'd simply become a bully myself.'

Susan was right. Although a desire for revenge is understandable, this kind of response helps neither child. For, while it is hard for parents and teachers to feel much sympathy for the bully, there is no doubt that bullies are just as much in need of help as their victims. For without assistance, aggressive children, who are often extremely anxious children, are unlikely to learn more socially acceptable ways of behaving. The idea that bullying is something children grow out of has been shown to be untrue. A long-term study of 800 American children revealed that children who bullied in first grade were very likely to grow up into aggressive, anti-social adults. Their marriages were less satisfactory and they were more likely to use violence against their own children. Their personal relationships were poor, they had fewer friends and stood a greater chance of getting into trouble with the law.

Children who never learn how to get along with others or join in their games, perhaps because they are the only child in the family, are especially at risk. Also vulnerable are youngsters with an obvious physical defect, such as a stammer, limp or visible birthmark. They can find themselves shunned by their playmates and singled out by the bully.

If you suspect that your child is being bullied or is prone to bullying, check the situation by ticking any of the statements below which apply.

My child:

1 is small for his/her age
2 cries easily
3 seldom joins in games
4 learns slowly
5 has a physical defect or disability
6 is an only child
7 prefers playing alone
8 tends to be withdrawn
9 lacks confidence
10 is rather unassertive
11 is big for his/her age
12 is very self-willed
13 always wants to be the centre of attention
14 is determined to get his/her own way
15 is rather aggressive
16 frequently gets spanked or smacked for misbehaviour
17 is frequently disobedient
18 often gets into trouble
19 does badly in school
20 has very few close friends

How to score

Total the ticks on statements 1–10, and then 11–20 separately. The first score indicates how vulnerable your child is to bullying. The second suggests the probability of him becoming a bully.

In each case, the higher the score, the greater the likelihood. 0–3: very low risk; 3–6: moderate risk; 7+: high risk. If your child scored 4 or more on statements 1–10 here are some practical steps to take.

If your child is bullied

Don't fall into the trap of encouraging your child to hit back, especially when this involves teaching him judo, karate or any other type of self-defence. You will simply be playing the bully at his own game. You cannot in the same breath condemn a child for attacking others while training your own child to hit back even harder.

Do help him or her to develop strong psychological defences, in order to withstand attempts at intimidation. Only by mastering these skills in childhood will he be able to withstand such adult forms of bullying as the sarcasm of superiors or the mockery of colleagues. Because children who fail to take a bully's bait make such poor victims their torment is usually quite short-lived.

Don't ridicule your child for not standing up for himself. This will only add to the anxiety, while undermining self-confidence still further.

Do encourage your child to learn a sport, not necessarily a team game. Any pursuit which offers both a challenge and the satisfaction of achievement is ideal. Especially valuable are sports in which your child takes on the elements – for instance, swimming, climbing, canoeing and sailing. These are particularly good at building confidence and self-esteem. A child who has successfully, and enjoyably, canoed down a fast-flowing river or climbed a steep rock-face is much less likely to be intimidated by a bullying older child. Needless to say, all such high-risk sports must be professionally taught and only done under expert supervision.

Do help your child make friends by keeping open house to them. A child who has many friends is less likely to become the victim of bullying.

Do try and persuade your child to see his would-be tormentors as weak and pathetic, rather than fierce and fearful. Once he starts to pity the bully rather than flinch from him, his power to scare your child has ended for ever.

Do use relaxation procedures and Mind Movies to strengthen assurance and resolve. Guide fantasies in which your child is confronted by a bully, but refuses to respond with either anxiety or aggression. Instead, he merely shrugs off the taunts and insults without feeling frightened or furious. Fearless Tiger can be used to bolster a younger child's self-confidence.

Don't immediately call on your child's teachers or the bully's parents to complain. For the sake of his self-esteem and future relationships with other children it is best, whenever possible, to allow your child to resolve matters for himself. Parental interventions, no matter how well intended, can make matters worse by having your child branded as a 'baby'. If your child is eight or older, only complain to teachers, or the bully's parents, when the bullying has gone on for some time or is getting more physically violent. If your child is younger than eight or slightly older but slightly built and easily scared you may feel it advisable to discuss the problem with his teachers at an earlier stage.

If your child is a bully

Bullies often copy the ways in which they see adults responding to a situation, so physical punishment only makes the problem worse. Children who are frequently smacked or slapped tend to use the same tactics on their smaller, more vulnerable, companions. So never beat children for bullying, however upset you are by their behaviour; it only makes them more willing to use aggression themselves.

Try to discover what social skills your child lacks that prevent him or her from playing amicably with others. Bullies are often incompetent children who cannot make an impression on their companions in any other way.

Bullying is especially upsetting because, whether a child is victim or aggressor one is left, feeling helpless and a bit guilty. After all, shouldn't a 'properly' raised child be either more willing to fight back or less aggressive in the first place? Such self-blame is neither helpful nor necessary. Bullying, and being bullied, is so common as to be almost a natural part of growing up, and does not necessarily imply any lasting defect of character. The best advice is to stay calm, avoid recriminations and approach the situation in a pragmatic – rather than a moralistic – manner.

Sixteen
Helping With Sexual Anxiety

Their child's sexual anxieties are among the most difficult and delicate problems parents ever have to deal with. One of the chief problems is that discussing the topic makes many adults extremely uncomfortable and anxious themselves. One mother told me that, although she prided herself on always talking openly and honestly to her fourteen-year-old daughter Carol-Ann, they had never been able to discuss sex. 'If she raises the subject I quickly change the subject,' Lynn explained. 'I become red with embarrassment.'

Lynn is not alone. A significant number of parents become so anxious when the topic arises that they hastily switch to a defensive mode. This may result in a refusal to talk about sexual activity at all (avoidance), the claim that sex education is best left to professional teachers (rationalisation) or that providing information will encourage promiscuity (projection or intellectualisation).

Some parents raise the same objections to the teaching of sex in school. In fact, research suggests that such education makes a child more, not less, responsible. In one study it was found that among adolescents who had not been given any sex education 31 per cent were sexually active. This compared with 17 per cent of teenagers who had received sex lessons at home and at school.

There is also a reluctance, on the part of many parents, to accept that their 'baby' has become a sexually mature adult. Coming to terms with the reality of their child's imminent departure from the nest arouses so much anxiety that parents often use denial of reality to protect themselves against it. Instead of dealing with their son or daughter on more equal terms, they attempt to force them to continue in the role of dependent and vulnerable child.

Even when parents see the wisdom of providing such guidance and teaching, their own upbringing and inhibitions may prevent them from doing so. Lynn's parents had taught her to consider sex as something respectable women never enjoyed and well-mannered people never mentioned. 'Now every time Carol-Ann raises the subject I curl up inside with shame,' she told me.

If you too have difficulty in talking about sex with your child, here are some practical suggestions for making these essential discussions easier to handle.

• Be certain of your facts before you start. Many parents have only the haziest knowledge of the biology or psychology of sex. And much of what they believe to be true is either misleading or downright wrong – a sad legacy of their own informal and ill-informed lessons behind the bicycle shed!

If you doubt this, check your own knowledge by ticking any of the statements below which you consider to be true:

1 Teenagers who have same-sex experiences grow up gay.
2 Regular masturbation is a threat to health.
3 An intact hymen is a sign of virginity.
4 Some people are naturally undersexed.
5 One's first sexual experience is the best.
6 You can catch VD from a lavatory seat.
7 Penis size is a good indication of sexual potency.
8 Girls are naturally less interested in sex than boys.
9 Impotence is a rare medical condition.
10 Some healthy women cannot experience orgasm.
11 You can catch AIDS by sharing a cup or glass.
12 Men do not possess a vagina. (Of all those statements this is one even well-educated adults most frequently get wrong. Men possess an organ called the *vagina*

masculina. During the earliest stage of development, the human embryo possesses a complete set of both male and female genitalia: gonads, which become either ovaries or testicles; genital swellings, the future labia major or scrotum; and the phallus, which develops into either a penis or clitoris. Once the final sex of the embryo has been determined, the unwanted organs fail to develop, although vestiges remain into adulthood. Men also have the equivalent of the hymen, the *seminal colliculus*, while women have a counterpart of the male's prostate in the Skenes glands, two small openings on either side of the urethra.)

How many of these statements did you tick as correct? Although all are widely believed, every one of them is false. If you ticked any of them, it might be advisable to read a sex education manual before offering guidance to your child.

• Never attempt to give formal sex lessons. There can be few more mutually embarrassing activities than to sit a child down and deliver a lecture on the 'facts of life'. This kind of instruction is better left to professional teachers in school. A far more helpful approach is to provide facts which your child hasn't yet been told in school, but is eager to find out, or which he or she may never learn from the somewhat mechanical approach taken by some sex-education teachers. By this I mean the role of sex as an important, but not necessarily central, part of a warm and loving relationship.

Take advantage of 'teaching opportunities', to convey information or offer guidance. Teaching opportunities are those moments when your child is eager to acquire knowledge and accept advice. They occur whenever he or she asks a question about sex, or makes a statement you know to be wrong.

• Answer all questions honestly, but reply in a way which suits the child's age, maturity and knowledge. A five-year-old who asks where babies come from can be told they are 'made in Mummy's tummy' without needing more anatomical details. A thirteen-year-old will certainly expect, and deserve, a more detailed explanation.

- Keeping pet rabbits or guinea pigs can be a useful way of introducing younger children to sexual reproduction. But do not be surprised if it takes them a while to appreciate that humans are made in the same way as baby rabbits!

- Start sex education early. Some parents believe there is no need to do so until puberty. In fact your child's sexual feelings, and curiosity, are well established by the age of two. Even at this age children can have vivid sexual fantasies and derive great pleasure from genital stimulation.

- Prepare your child for puberty by providing clear, factual information about what to expect. Parents are usually far better at doing this with their daughters, who generally know what to expect when they start menstruating, then they are with their sons. Many boys are shocked and horrified the first time they produce sperm, because they had no idea what to expect or understanding of what is happening.

Factual information, presented in a matter-of-fact way, especially prior to these physical events, will do much to reduce the anxiety many teenagers suffer as a result of these natural functions.

Do not leave such instructions too late. Although, on average, a boy has his first ejaculation at around fourteen and girls begin menstruating at thirteen, there are, as the table below shows, wide variations. Boys as young as six have been known to ejaculate, while others may not do so until late in their teens.

AVERAGE ages at which different stages of puberty occur		
	Boys	Girls
Pubic hair appears	13.5	12.3
Growth spurt starts/ends	14.5–17.8	12.8–15.8
Voice breaks	14.4	–
First ejaculation	13.9	–
First menstrual period	–	13.0
Breasts develop	–	12.4

Production of sperm in a boy and ova in a girl marks the end of puberty and the onset of adolescence.

- When talking to your child use the correct terms rather than taking refuge in euphemism, which are often anxiety-arousing; e.g. talk about menstruation or periods rather than 'the curse'. One girl who wasn't at all worried when she started her menstrual periods lived for years in dread of the 'curse' her mother had warned her to expect. It was some time before she realised that her mother did not mean that she was the victim of witchcraft!

- Place sexual activity in context. Studies suggest that, while sex is an important factor, it comes well behind commitment, affection, sharing, talking openly and having a sense of humour as a factor in sustaining a long and loving relationship.

Although many aspects of sex make children anxious, my experience suggests that there are two topics which cause so much embarrassment to youngsters they are rarely willing to reveal them to parents. Even when the relationship is one of trust and affection.

Anxiety over public nudity

Soon after he started senior school, Caroline noticed that her thirteen-year-old son John had begun to hate sports. On days when gym or games were on the timetable, he often complained of feeling ill and pleaded for a sick note. But it was only after he started to play truant on sports afternoons that Caroline discovered the true reason why her son so disliked games. What upset him was having to take a communal shower afterwards. He felt embarrassed by and ashamed of his body, and fearful of being ridiculed.

Although the boy's reaction was more extreme than most, his anxiety over having to shower in public is far from rare. A significant number of children, especially those in their early teens, are upset at appearing naked in front of others. Is your own child among them? He or she could be without you realising it, since this is the type of anxiety which children usually feel too embarrassed to discuss. Here are some of the signs to watch for; tick any which apply.

My child:

- Always locks the door when taking a bath.
- Is angry if I enter his/her bedroom without first knocking.
- Is careful to keep covered up when changing on the beach.
- Uses a private changing cubicle at swimming baths.
- Hates sharing a bedroom with another child.
- Dislikes medical examinations which involve undressing.
- Is upset by nudity on TV.
- Makes disparaging jokes about his/her body.
- Tries to avoid showering at school.
- Is embarrassed at seeing same-sex friends undressed.

If you ticked more than five statements, it's likely that your child is made anxious by nudity. There are three main reasons why this may be so.

1: An emotional need for privacy
As parents of teenagers well know, they can guard their privacy very jealously. Any trespass on their territory, whether it is going unannounced into their bedroom or borrowing an item of personal property without asking, can trigger a furious outburst. Being compelled to undress in public, an extreme violation of their emotional need for privacy, can also cause severe emotional conflict and resentment.

2: Concern about supposed imperfections
Adolescents often have an exaggerated concern about physical imperfections, such as a spotty back, fat legs or flat chest. Being forced to reveal these imagined failings can make even a well-adjusted boy or girl feel extremely anxious.

3: Worry that they are sexually inadequate
This stems from the very different rates at which children mature. Penis and breast size are particular causes for concern, making the less developed child feel inferior. The American comedian Woody Allen has joked that Freud was wrong in claiming that only girls suffer from penis envy. And,

like many of his jests, it contains more than a grain of truth. Adolescent boys can feel extremely anxious if they regard their penis as smaller or thinner than those of same-age companions.

When, as sometimes happens, PE teachers shower at the same time, to show they are 'one of the boys', comparisons between adult genitalia and their less developed organs can lead boys to feel inadequate and anxious. The often overtly sexual teasing, mockery and homo-erotic horseplay which occurs in many all-male changing-rooms only makes their agony more intense.

Similarly, girls will suffer agonies of anxiety and despair because their breasts are not as large or shapely as those of their friends, or because they are overdeveloped for their age. They can readily convince themselves that no boy will ever find them attractive unless their bust develops more fully. And this self-imposed belief in inevitable rejection leads to high levels of anxiety.

If public nudity causes difficulties for your child, here are six practical ways to help.

Don't ask the school to excuse your child from showering after games or PE. This will only make him 'different' from the others and so an even more likely target for ridicule.

Do always respect your child's privacy. Even if you have no objections to him or her seeing you naked around the house, be prepared to accept that it causes them embarrassment. A teenager's bedroom should be off-limits to all other members of the family except with his or her permission. The same applies to the bathroom when he or she is in there.

Do understand and accept his or her new-found modesty. If you have always brought your child up to feel no shame about nudity, this sudden shyness may be difficult for you to take seriously. But you must recognise the desire to remain covered in company as a perfectly reasonable and legitimate right. Making jokes at their expense, or telling them that they are being silly, will only heighten anxiety.

Do make sure your child understands the 'facts of life'. Great anxiety is often based on just a little ignorance. If you suspect that lack of knowledge, or misinformation, is causing the difficulties, explain the basics of sexual development as clearly and simply as possible (see above). Emphasise that, just as some people are taller or shorter than others, so too there are differences in the size of breasts or penis, and the extent of pubic hair. Make it plain that genital size does not reflect on potency, sexual prowess or attractiveness.

Do reassure your child that a same-sex attraction is nothing to feel anxious or guilty about (see below).

Do enhance your child's self-confidence by allowing increased independence. Let him or her make decisions about the choice of clothes, bedroom décor and so on. Encourage active participation in family decision-making, but when doing so be prepared to give serious attention to their ideas and views. The more independent and self-assured a child feels the less likely he or she is to become upset by nudity – or indeed by other common causes of anxiety.

Anxiety over same-sex attraction

Many, probably the majority, of teenagers have homosexual inclinations. By this I simply mean an erotic attraction to their own sex (*homo* comes from the Greek *homeo*, not from the Latin word for man, and means 'similar to' or 'the same as'). In the early 1950s, the American researcher Kinsey aroused a storm of protest with his suggestion that, far from being a rare aberration, same-sex experiences during adolescence are relatively common.

In pre- and early adolescent boys contempt of girls, being a member of a gang and hero-worshipping males is commonplace. So too is learning or observing how to masturbate. During horseplay in changing-rooms and showers it is far from uncommon for boys to touch and manipulate each other, frequently to the point of ejaculation.

Such activities, comment Philip Cauthery and Martin Cole,*

> paradoxically mark the start of the process by which the young male frees himself from the sexual restraints and

---

*The Fundamentals of Sex, W.H. Allen, 1971.

fears of his relationship with his mother and begins to assume his adult sexual and masculine role which will eventually allow him to love, and make love to, another woman.

Girls, from around the age of eight onwards, commonly have intense 'crushes' on other girls or women, are interested in looking at female nudes and, in adolescence, either fantasise or indulge in sexual games with other girls.

Although many adults look back on their same-sex adolescent experiences with guilt, and the fear that it implies a latent homosexuality, such behaviour is so widespread that it must be considered natural rather than any form of aberration. The same applies to homoerotic dreams, and even sexual arousal – partial erection or vaginal lubrication – when viewing, or fantasising about, people of the same sex. The only problem which arises from such experiences is the unnecessary anxiety, depression and guilt which they arouse.

Children are seldom sufficiently confident of their parents to confide such feelings to them, but if your child does you should regard it is a considerable compliment. You have inspired such trust in them that they are willing to discuss what is probably the most sensitive and painful of all adolescent anxieties. On no account must you betray that trust by appearing shocked or critical, by refusing to listen or talk about the subject further, by condemnation or by outraged disgust. Even if you are upset by such disclosures, and there is absolutely no good reason to be distressed, remain outwardly calm and non-judgemental. Reassure your child that, as I have explained, these experiences are universal. They certainly do not mean that homosexuality will continue to be their chosen sexual orientation.

Although sexual anxieties can make a child's life utterly miserable, and continue to haunt them into adulthood if left unresolved, removing such fears is often remarkably straightforward. In no other area of anxiety does factual information, delivered in a calm, neutral and non-judgemental manner, prove so effective an antidote.

Correcting misapprehensions or misunderstandings may be all that is needed to free your child from a previously crushing burden of guilt and fear.

Part Five
Living without anxiety

Seventeen
Living Without Anxiety

Sometimes anxieties or fears disappear almost overnight as a result of using the procedures which I have described. The mother of one nine-year-old boy told me how, after her child had learned to use Floppy Bear and Fearless Tiger in class, his attitude towards school was transformed. Anxiety vanished and he became far more positive and confident about his work. Just having those two images to turn to whenever he started feeling apprehensive gave him such a sense of control that his whole outlook changed.

Often, too, correcting a piece of misinformation is enough to banish anxiety. An eight-year-old became terrified after his teacher had told him he was 'ignorant'. Why? Because her comment came at a time when a campaign warning of the dangers of AIDS was promoting the slogan, 'Don't Die of Ignorance'. He was convinced that, since he was 'ignorant', he was going to die. Although that fear had festered away for weeks, and made him extremely distressed, it took only five minutes of calm explanation to put matters right once the cause of his terror had been identified.

The rapid removal of a deeply entrenched anxiety, phobia or fear tends, however, to be the exception rather than the rule. In most cases you are not going to see an instant transformation of a fearful child into a fearless one. The usual course is a gradual one, with your child slowly gaining in confidence and assurance as he, or she, becomes increasingly willing to tackle a previously avoided activity.

There will also be setbacks and disappointments along the way. Just when you felt sure that your child was making excellent progress along the road to a fear-free lifestyle, there may be an unexpected regression. He will suddenly, and for no reason either of you can discover, panic. She will abruptly refuse to tackle some activity which, only a few days earlier, was causing no more than mild apprehension.

Be prepared for such temporary reversals and do not allow them to discourage either you or your child. When removing an anxiety, especially one which has been causing trouble for some time, it is quite normal for progress to fluctuate. In fact, this is what happens whenever we master any new skill. Think back to the time when you learned to drive and you may remember that on one day you could handle the car pretty well, but on the very next lesson regressed and drove like a rank beginner all over again. A reassuring image to hold in mind is that of a person walking steadily up a flight of stairs with a yo-yo in one hand. If you watch the rise and fall of the yo-yo it may not appear that any gains are being made. But if, instead, you switch your attention to the person climbing the stairs you will see that he is, slowly but surely, nearing his target.

A child who has been anxious for many months is very good at feeling anxiety. After all, he or she has been practising day in and day out for many weeks. If you do anything regularly for that length of time you are bound to become proficient at it. Anxious, phobic or fearful children are often extremely good at working themselves into a highly anxious state. As we saw in the early chapters, a small increase in physical arousal can trigger negative mental thoughts and ideas about not being able to cope. These, in turn, cause the body to become more aroused, the heart to beat more rapidly, the stomach to churn, muscles to tense, and so on. Breaking this vicious circle takes effort and enthusiasm.

During this time your child will need constant encouragement to continue. Do not become discouraged yourself, even when the process of eliminating anxiety seems to be taking far longer than you had hoped or expected. Never mock the child for being weak or silly, as, far from shocking them into a more positive frame of mind, as some parents seem to believe, it only deepens the anxiety and makes it even more intractable.

You should also realise that anxiety can serve a positive purpose in the child's life, which means that when it is given up there could well be a gap left behind. For instance, a child who is afraid of school and plays truant probably finds sneaking back home to watch TV or hanging around amusement arcades is far more interesting than what goes on in the classroom. So he is not only being rewarded for his avoidance by feeling far less anxious, but also by having a more stimulating day to look forward to. Similarly, a child whose anxiety has made adults very sympathetic and understanding could be reluctant to give it up for fear that more demands will be made on her.

This means that at the same time as working to remove anxieties, you must try and build in compensations for the benefits which will no longer be available once the fears have been dealt with.

In the case of the school phobic, for instance, try and encourage an interest in school-centred activities which would have appeal, such as playing sports, joining the drama group, electronics society or chess club. One fifteen-year-old changed his mind about school when he was able to join a motor engineering society started by the technical department. The school acquired some old bangers which the boys were shown how to repair and maintain. This boy not only began attending school regularly, in order to be allowed to join the society, but also improved greatly in the maths and science classes as he came to realise that these previously abstract subjects had very practical uses.

Anxious children generally have a poor self-image. They regard themselves as weak, submissive and underachieving in many, if not all, areas of their lives. This does not mean, as I have already explained, that they really are underachievers; indeed, they may be doing extremely well in class. What matters is the goals they set themselves and the targets they feel others expect them to achieve. Where parents are over perfectionist and constantly critical, anxiety levels even in high-flyers are likely to be very high.

Give your child as much responsibility and independence as possible. Help boost self-esteem by praising successes and dealing with setbacks in a neutral manner. 'Ear-shotting' is an excellent way of giving your child's esteem a real boost. Here, instead of saying how pleased you are straight to his face you allow him to overhear a positive comment made to your partner. For instance, when your child is in a nearby room, but able to hear what you say, tell your partner: 'I was so impressed by the way John did . . .' and describe, briefly, what happened.

Ear-shotting needs to be done carefully in order to sound convincing, but when it works it often proves even more effective than direct praise. After all, we all tend to believe that people are more polite to our faces than they are behind our backs. This gives the positive comment, seemingly overheard by accident, even greater credibility and potency.

Finally, to make this home-help plan for overcoming anxiety enjoy the greatest chance of success, follow these four P's.

- Be Positive – assume that the plan is going to work. Believe it is going to work, and it will work. If doubtful, try the procedures for yourself before using them with your child. This is especially important if you are anxious or fearful yourself. Not only will it assist in bringing your own anxieties under control, but it will give you practical experience of the power these procedures possess.
- Be Patient – do not assume that anxiety will vanish rapidly, or that your child will immediately adopt the procedures suggested. As I have said, anxiety can have positive benefits for a child which may make him or her resist its removal.
- Be Persistent – keep working at the procedures and do not abandon them if immediate progress is not forthcoming. Remember that chronic anxiety has been practised over a long period of time, which means it will also take time to remove.
- Be Prudent – know when to push and when to relax the pressure. Never force your child to take a step for which they are not ready. If excessive anxiety is being experienced, your child is attempting something too hard.

Anxiety is a curse which can cast a damning spell over your child's life. But there is a cure. It is to be found in this book – and in your hands.

Bibliography

Ackerman, N. W. *The Psychodynamics of Family Life*, New York, Macmillan, 1958

Agras, W. S. 'Transfer during systematic desensitization therapy', *Behaviour Research and Therapy*, 5 (1967), pp. 193–270

Agras, W. S., Chapin, H. N. and Oliveau, D.C. 'The natural history of phobia', *Archives of General Psychiatry*, 26 (1972), pp. 315–17

Agras, W. S. Leitenberg, H. and Barlow, D. H. 'Social reinforcement in the modification of agoraphobia', *Archives of General Psychiatry* (1968), pp. 423–7

Agras, S., Sylvester, D., and Oliveau, D. 'The epidemiology of common fears and phobias', *Comprehensive Psychiatry*, 10 (1969), pp. 151–6

Aitkin, R. C. B. and Zealley, A. K. 'The measurement of moods', *British Journal of Hospital Medicine* (1970), pp. 215–24

Akiskal, H. S. and McKinney, W. T. 'Depressive disorders: towards a unified hypothesis', *Science*, 182 (1973), pp. 20–8

Altrocchi, J. *Abnormal Behaviour*, New York, Harcourt Brace Jovanovich, 1980

Andrews, J. D. W. 'Psychotherapy of Phobias', *Psychological Bulletin*, 66 (1966), pp. 455–80

Arieti, S. 'New views on the psychodynamics of phobias', *American Journal of Psychotherapy*, 33 (1979), pp. 82–95

Averill, J. R. 'Personal control over aversive stimuli and its relationship to stress', *Psychological Bulletin*, 80 (1973), pp. 286–303

Bandura, A., Blanchard, E.G. and Ritter, B. 'Relative efficacy of desensitization and modelling approaches for inducing behavioural, affective and attitudinal changes', *Journal of Personality and Social Psychology*, 13 (1969), No. 3, pp. 173–99

Barker, R.C. *Adjustment to Physical Handicap and Illness*, New York, McGraw-Hill, 1953

Barlow, D. H., Leitenberg, H., Agras, W.S. and Wincze, J.P. 'The transfer gap in systematic desensitization: An analogue study', *Behaviour Research and Therapy*, 7 (1969), pp. 191–6

Barlow, D. H., Leitenberg, H., Agras, W. S. and Wincze, J. P. 'An experimental analysis of the effectiveness of shaping in reducing maladaptive avoidance behaviour: an analogue study', *Behaviour Research and Therapy*, 7 (1970), pp. 165–73

Bauer, D. H. 'An explanatory study of developmental changes in children's fears', *Journal of Child Development and Psychiatry*, 17 (1976), pp. 69–74

Beck, A.T., Laude, R. and Bohnert, M. 'Ideational components of anxiety neurosis', *Archives of General Psychiatry*, 31 (1974), pp. 319–25

Beck, A.T. and Rush, A. J. 'A cognitive model of anxiety formation and anxiety resolution', in I. Sarason and C. Spielberger (eds), *Stress and Anxiety*, vol. 2, New York, Halsted Press, 1975

Benjamin, S., Marks, I. M. and Huson, J. 'The role of active muscular desensitization', *Psychological Medicine*, 2 (1972), pp. 381–90

Burns, L. E. and Thorpe, G. L. 'The epidemiology of fears and phobias with particular reference to the national survey of agoraphobics', *Journal of International Medical Research*, 5 (1977a), Supplement (5), pp. 1–7

Burns, L. E. and Thorpe, G. L. 'Fears and clinical phobias: epidemiological aspects and the national survey of agoraphobics', *Journal of Internal Medical Research* (1977b), Supplement (1), pp. 132–9

Cohen, J. *Behaviour in Uncertainty*, London, George Allen and Unwin, 1964

Cook, S. W. 'A survey of methods used to produce "experimental neurosis"', *American Journal of Psychiatry*, 95 (1939), pp. 1259–76

DiLoreto, A. *Comparative Psychotherapy*, New York, Aldine-Atherton, 1971

Dinnerstein, D. *The Rocking of the Cradle and the Ruling of the World*, London, Souvenir Press, 1976

Dixon, J. J., de Monchaux, C. and Sandler, J. 'Patterns of anxiety: An analysis of social anxieties', *British Journal of Medical Psychology*, 30 (1957), pp. 34–40

Eme, R. and Schmidt, D. 'The stability of children's fears', *Child Development*, 49 (1978), pp. 1277–9

Emerson, E. and Lucas, H. 'Preparedness and the development of aversive associations', *British Journal of Clinical Psychology*, 20 (1981), pp. 293–4

Emmelkamp, P. M. G. 'The behavioural study of clinical phobias', in Herson M., Eisler, R. M. and Miller, P. M. (eds) *Progress in Behaviour Modification*, vol. 8 (1979), pp. 55–125

Emmelkamp, P. M. G. and Emmelkamp-Bender, A. 'Effects of historically portrayed modeling and group treatment on self-observation: A comparison with agoraphobics', *Behaviour Research and Therapy*, 13 (1975), pp. 135–9

Emmelkamp, P. M. G., Kuipers, A. C. M. and Eggeraal, J. B. 'Cognitive modification versus prolonged exposure in vivo: A comparison with agoraphobics as subjects', *Behaviour Research and Therapy*, 16 (1978), pp. 34–41

Emmelkamp, P. M. G. and Ultee, K. A. 'A comparison of successive approximation and self-observation in the treatment of agoraphobia', *Behaviour Therapy*, 5 (1974), (5) pp. 606–13

Emmelkamp, P. M. G. and Wessels, H. 'Flooding in imagination v. flooding in vivo: a comparison with agoraphobics', *Behaviour Research and Therapy*, 13 (1975), pp. 7–15

Erwin, W. J. 'Confinement in the production of human neurosis: The barber's chair syndrome', *Behaviour Research and Therapy*, 1 (1963), pp. 175–83

Eysenck, H. J. *Behaviour Therapy and the Neuroses*, New York, Pergamon, 1963

Eysenck, H. J. 'Learning theory and behaviour therapy', *Journal of Mental Science*, 105 (1963), pp. 61–75

Eysenck, H. J. *The Biological Basis of Personality*, Illinois, Charles C. Thomas, 1977

Eysenck, H. J. 'A conditioning model of neurosis', *Behavioural and Brain Sciences*, 2 (1979), pp. 155–99

Fehrenbach, P. A. and Thelen, M. H. 'Behavioural approaches to the treatment of aggressive disorders', *Behaviour Modification*, 6, 4 (1982), pp. 465–97

Fischer, W. F. *Theories of Anxiety*, London, Harper and Row, 1970

Foa, E. B. and Emmelkamp, P. M. G. *Failures in Behaviour Therapy*, New York, Wiley, 1983

Fodor, I. G. 'The phobic syndrome in women: Implications for treatment', in Franks, V. and Burtle, V. (eds) *Women in Therapy: New Psychotherapies for a Changing Society*, New York, Brunner/Manzel, 1974

Fodor, I. *Phobias in Women: Therapeutic Approaches*, New York, BMA Audio Cassette Publications, 1978

Fogarty, M., Rapoport, R. and Rapoport, R. N. *Sex, Career and Family*, London, George Allen and Unwin, 1971

Foulds, G. A. *Personality and Personal Illness*, London, Tavistock, 1965

Frankel, F. H. and Orne, M. T. 'Hypnotisability and phobic behaviour, *Archives of General Psychiatry*, 33 (1976), pp. 1259–61

Freud, S. 'The Neuro-Psychoses of Defence: (An attempt at a psychological theory of acquired hysteria, of many phobias and obsessions and of certain hallucinatory psychoses', (1894), in *Standard edition of the complete psychological works of Sigmund Freud*, London, Hogarth Press, 1962

Freud, S. 'Analysis of a phobia in a 5-year-old boy', (1909), in

Standard Edition (vol. 3.) London, Hogarth Press, 1962

Freud, S. 'Turnings in the ways of psychoanalytic therapy', (1919), reprinted as Chapter 34 in *Standard Edition*, (Vol. 2.), London, Hogarth Press, 1962

Freud, S. 'Inhibition, symptoms and anxiety', (1926), in *Standard Edition*, London, Hogarth Press, 1962

Friedman, J. H. 'Short-term psychotherapy of "phobia of travel"', *American Journal of Psychotherapy*, New York, John Wiley, 1950

Fry, W. F. 'The marital context of anxiety syndrome', *Family Process*, 1 (1962), pp. 245–52

Furst, J. B. and Cooper, A. 'Combined use of imaginal and interoceptive stimuli in desensitizing fear of heart attacks', *Journal of Behaviour Therapy and Experimental Psychology*, (1970), pp. 87–9

Gara, M. A., 'Back to basics in personality study – the individual person's own organisation of experience', in Mancuso, J. C. and Adams-Webber, J. R. (eds) *The Construing Person*, New York, Praeger, 1982

Gatchell, R. J. and Gaas, E. 'Effects of arousal level on short and long term habituation of orienting response', *Physiological Psychology*, 4 (1976), pp. 66–8

Geer, J. H. 'Development of a scale to measure fear', *Behaviour Research and Therapy*, 3 (1965), pp. 45–53

Gelder, M. G., Bancroft, J. H. J., Gath, D. H., Johnston, D. W., Mathews, A. M. and Shaw, P. M. 'Specific and non-specific factors in behaviour therapy', *British Journal of Psychiatry*, 123 (1973), pp. 445–62

Gelder, M. G., Marks, I. M., and Wolff, H. H. 'Desensitization and psychotherapy in the treatment of phobic states: a controlled enquiry', *British Journal of Psychiatry*, 113 (1967), pp. 53–73

Gittelman, R. (ed.) *Anxiety Disorders of Childhood*, New York, The Guildford Press, 1986

Goffman, E. 'Stigma: Notes on the management of spoiled identity', Englewood Cliffs, NJ, Prentice Hall, 1963

Goldberg, L. and Breznitz, S. *Handbook of Stress*, New York, Free Press, 1982

Gove, W. R. and Tudor, J. F. 'Adult sex roles and mental illness', *American Journal of Sociology*, 78 (1973), pp. 812–35

Graziano, A. M. (ed.) *Behaviour Therapy With Children II*, Chicago, Aldine, 1975

Gray J. A. *The Psychology of Fear and Stress*, London, Weidenfeld and Nicholson, 1971

Gray, J. A. *The Neuropsychology of Anxiety*, Oxford, Oxford University Press, 1983

Greer, S. 'The prognosis of anxiety states', in M. H. Lader (ed.) Studies of Anxiety, *British Journal of Psychiatry Special Publication* No. 3, 1969

Grings, W. W. 'Orientation, conditioning and learning', *Psychophysiology*, 14 (1977), pp. 343–50

Gurland, P. J., Yorkeston, N. J. and Goldberg, K. 'The structured and scaled interview to assess maladjustment: Description, rationale, development, factor analysis, reliability and validity', *Archives of General Psychiatry*, 27 (1978), pp. 259–67

Hall-Smith, P. and Ryle, A. 'Marital patterns, hostility and personal illness', *British Journal of Psychiatry*, 115 (1969), pp. 1197–8

Hamilton, M. 'Standardised assessment and recording of depressive symptoms', *Psychiatrica Neurologia and Neurochirurgia*, 72 (1969), pp. 201–5

Hayden, B. C. 'Experience – a case for possible change: the modulation corollary', in Mancuso, J. C. and Adams-Webber, J. R. (eds) *The Construing Person*, New York, Praeger, 1982

Head, H. *Studies in Neurology* (vol. 2.), London, Hodder and Stoughton, 1920

Heikkinen, C. A. 'Another look at teaching experience and closed-mindedness', *Journal of Counselling Psychology*, 22 (1975), pp. 79–83

Hensen, M. 'Self assessment of fear', *Behaviour Therapy*, 4 (1973), pp. 241–57

Hensen, M. and Bellack, A. S. *Behavioural Assessment: A Practical Handbook*, Oxford, Pergamon Press, 1976

Hilgard, E. R. and Bower, G. H. *Theories of Learning*, Englewood Cliffs, New Jersey, Prentice-Hall, 1975

Hinchcliffe, M. K., Vaughan, P. W., Hooper, D. and Roberts, F. J. 'The melancholy marriage: An inquiry into the interaction of depression. II Expressiveness', *British Journal Medical Psychology*, 50 (2) (1977), pp. 125–42

Hollingshead, A. B. and Redlich, F. C. *Social Class and Mental Illness*, New York, John Wiley, 1958

Holmes, K. 'Phobia and counterphobia: family aspects of agoraphobia', *Journal Family Therapy*, 4 (1982), pp. 133–52

Holt, J. *How Children Fail*, Harmondsworth, Penguin Books, 1977

Horder, J. and Horder, C. 'Illness and General Practice', *The Practitioner*, p. 193, 1954

Horney, K. *Self-Analysis*, London, Routledge and Kegan Paul, 1942

Hugdahl, K., Fredrikson, M. and Ohman, A. 'Preparedness and arousability as determinants of electrodermal conditioning', *Behaviour Research and Therapy*, 15 (1977), pp. 315–53

Jacobson, E. *Progressive Relaxation*, Chicago, University of Chicago Press, 1938

Janis, I. L. and Mann, L. *Decision Making A Psychological Analysis of Conflict, Choice, and Commitment*, New York, The Free Press, 1977

Jerslid, A. T. and Holmes, F. B. *Children's Fears*, New York, Columbia University, 1935

Kartsounis, L. D. and Pickersgill, M. J. 'Orienting responses to stimuli others fear', *British Journal of Clinical Psychology*, 20 (1981), pp. 261–73

Katkin, E. S. and Silver-Hoffmann, L. S. 'Sex differences and self-report of fear: a psychophysiological assessment', *Journal Abnormal Psychology*, 85 (1976), pp. 607–10

Katz, J. M. 'Discrepancy, arousal and labelling: towards a psychosocial theory of emotion', paper presented to the World Congress of Sociology, Uppsala, Sweden, August, 1978

Kazdin, A. E. and Wilcoxon, L. A. 'Systematic desensitization and non-specific treatment effects: A methodological evaluation', *Psychological Bulletin*, 83 (1976), pp. 729–58

Kellner, R. and Sheffield, B. F. 'A self-rating scale for distress', *Psychological Medicine*, 3 (1973), pp. 88–101

Kessel, N. and Shepherd, M. 'The health and attitudes of people who seldom consult a doctor', *Medical Care*, 3 pp. 6–10, 1965

Kirschenbaum, D. S., Dielman, J. S. and Karoly, P. 'Efficacy of behavioural contracting: target behaviours, performance criteria and settings', *Behaviour Modification*, (Vol. 6.) 4 (1982), pp. 499–518

Lacey, J. I. 'Somatic response patterning and stress: Some revisions of activation theory', in Appley, M. H. and Trumbull, R. (eds) *Psychological Stress: Issues in Research*, New York, Appleton Century Crofts, 1967

Lader, M. H. 'Predictive value of autonomic measures in patients with phobic states', DPM dissertation, University of London, 1966

Lader, M. H., Gelder, M. G. and Marks, I. 'Palmar skin-conductance measures as predictors of response to desensitization', *Journal of Psychosomatic Research*, 11 (1967), pp. 283–90

Lader, M. H. and Mathews, A. M. 'A physiological model of phobic anxiety and desensitization', *Behaviour Research and Therapy*, 6 (1968), pp. 411–21

Landfield, A. W. 'Meaningfulness of self, ideal and other as related to own versus therapist's personal construct dimensions', *Psychological Reports*, 16 (1965), pp. 605–8

Landfield, A. W. 'Interpretive man. The enlarged self-image', in Landfield, A. W. (ed.) *Nebraska Symposium on Motivation. Personal Construct Psychology*, Nebraska, 1977

Lang, P. J. 'Fear reduction and fear behaviour: problems in treating a construct', in Shlien, J. M. (ed.) *Research in Psychotherapy*, (Vol. 3),

Washington DC, American Psychological Association, 1968

Lang, P. J. 'The mechanics of desensitization and the laboratory study of fear', in Franks C. M. (ed.) *Behaviour Therapy Appraisal and Status*, New York, McGraw Hill, 1969

Lang, P. J. 'The application of psychophysiological methods to the study of psychotherapy and behaviour modification', in Bergin, A. E. and Garfield, S. L. (eds) *Handbook of Psychotherapy and Behaviour Change: An Empirical Analysis*, New York, Wiley, 1971

Lang, P. J., Lazovik, A. and Reynolds, D. 'Desensitization, suggestibility and pseudotherapy', *Journal Abnormal Psychology*, 70 (1966), pp. 395–402

Lahey, B. B. and Kazdin, A. E. (eds) *Advances in Clinical Child Psychology*, New York, Plenum Press, 1977

Lapouse, T. and Monk, M. A. 'Fears and worries of a representative sample of children', *American Journal of Orthopsychiatry*, 29 (1959), pp. 803–18

Lazarus, A. A. *Behaviour Therapy And Beyond*, New York, McGraw-Hill Book Company, 1971

Lazarus, M., 'Mathophobia: Some personal speculations', *The Principal*, Jan/Feb (1974), p. 18

Lazarus, R. S. 'Emotions and adaptation: Conceptual and empirical relations', *Nebraska Symposium on Motivation*, 16 (1968), pp. 175–266

Lazarus, R. S., Averill, J. R. and Opton, E. M. Jr. 'The psychology of coping: Issues in research and assessment', in Coelho, C. V., Hamburg, D. H. and Adams, J. E. (eds) *Coping and Adaptation*, New York, Basic Books, 1974

Leitner, L. M. 'Literalism, perspectivism, chaotic fragmentalism and psychotherapy techniques', *British Journal Medical Psychology*, 55 (1982), pp. 307–17

Lewis, D. *The Secret Language of Your Child*, London, Souvenir Press, 1978

Lewis, D. *How To Be A Gifted Parent*, London, Souvenir Press, 1979

Lewis, D. *You Can Teach Your Child Intelligence*, London, Souvenir Press, 1982

Lewis, D. *Fight Your Phobia And Win*, London, Sheldon Press, 1985

Lewis, D. *The Alpha Plan*, London, Methuen, 1986

Lewis, D. *Mind Skills*, London, Souvenir Press, 1987

Lewis, D. and Greene, J. *Thinking Better*, New York, Holt, Reinhart and Winston, 1982

Lewis, D. and Greene, J. *Know Your Own Mind*, New York, Rawson Associates, 1983

Lewis D. and Greene, J. *Your Child's Drawings . . . Their Hidden Meaning*, London, Hutchinson, 1983

Lick, J. and Bootzin, R. 'Expectancy factors in the treatment of fear: Methodological and theoretical issues', *Psychological Bulletin*, 82 (1975), (6), pp. 917–31

Lick, J. 'Expectation, false galvanic skin response feedback and systematic desensitization in the modification of phobic behaviour', *Journal of Consulting and Clinical Psychology*, 43 (1975), pp. 557–67

Lief, H. I. 'Anxiety reaction', in Freedman, A. M. and Kaplan, H. I. (eds) *Comprehensive Textbook of Psychiatry*, Baltimore, Williams and Wilkins, 1967

Litman, T. J. 'The Family as a Basic Unit in Health and Medical Care', *Social Science and Medicine*, 8 (1974), pp. 495–519

Lowenthal, M. F., Thurnher, M. and Chiriboga, D. *Four Stages of Life: A Comparative Study of Women and Men Facing Transitions*, San Francisco, Jossey-Bass, 1975

Lubonsky, L., Auerbach. A. H. et al 'Factors influencing the outcome of psychotherapy', *Psychological Bulletin*, 75 (1971), pp. 145–85

Lum, L. C. in Hill, O. (ed.) *Modern Trends In Psychosomatic Medicine*, (Vol. 3), London, Butterworth, p. 196, 1976

Maurer, A. 'What children fear', *Journal of Genetic Psychology*, 106 (1956), pp. 265–77

MacFarlane, J. W., Allen, L. and Honzik, M. P. *A developmental study of the behaviour problems of normal children between twenty-one months and fourteen years*, Berkeley, University of California Press, 1954

Marks, I. M. *Fears and Phobias*, New York, Academic Press, 1969

Marks, I. M. 'The classification of phobic disorder', *British Journal of Psychiatry*, 116 (1970), pp. 377–86

Marks, I. M. 'Phobic disorders four years after treatment: A prospective follow-up, *British Journal of Psychiatry*, 118 (1971), pp. 683–8

Marks, I. M. 'Reduction of fear: Towards a unifying theory', paper presented at the Joint Meeting of the Canadian Psychiatric Association, June 1972, 1973

Marks, I. M., Boulougouris, J. and Marset, P. 'Flooding versus desensitization in the treatment of phobic patients: a crossover study', *British Journal of Psychiatry*, 119 (1971), pp. 353–75

Marks, I. M. and Gelder, M. G. 'A controlled retrospective study of behaviour therapy in phobic patients', *British Journal of Psychiatry*, 111 (1965), pp. 561–73

Marks, I. M. and Gelder, M. G. 'Different ages of onset in varieties of phobia', *American Journal of Psychiatry*, 123 (1966), pp. 218–21

Marks, I. M., Gelder, M. G. and Edwards, G. 'Hypnosis and desensitization for phobics: A controlled prospective trial' *British Journal of Psychiatry*, 114 (1968), pp. 1263–74

Marks, I. M. and Lader M. 'Anxiety states (anxiety neurosis): A review', *Journal of Nervous and Mental Diseases*, 156 (1973), pp. 3–18

Marks, I. M., Marset, P., Boulougouris. J. and Hudson, J. 'Physiological accompaniments of neutral and phobic imagery', *Psychological Medicine*, 1 (1971), pp. 299–307

Marks, I. M. and Mathews, A. M. 'Brief standard self-rating for phobic patients', *Behaviour Therapy And Research*, 17 (1979), pp. 263–7

Marzagao, K. R. 'Systematic desensitization treatment of kleptomania', *Journal of Behaviour Therapy and Experimental Psychiatry*, 3 (1972), pp. 327–8

Mather, M. D. and Degun, G. S. 'A comparative study of hypnosis and relaxation', *British Journal Medical Psychology*, 48 (1975), pp. 55–63

Mathews, A. 'Specific and non-specific factors in behaviour therapy', paper presented at the Third Annual Conference of the Behavioural Engineering Association, Wexford, Ireland, 1971

Mathews, A. M., Johnston, D. S., Shaw, P. M. and Gelder, M. G. 'Process variables and the prediction of outcome in behaviour therapy', *British Journal of Psychiatry* 123 (1974), pp. 445–62

Mathews A. M. and Shaw, P. 'Emotional arousal and persuasion effects in flooding', *Behaviour Research and Therapy*, 11 (1973), pp. 587–98

McNamara, J. R. and Blumer, C. A. 'Role playing to assess social competence: Ecological validity considerations', *Behaviour Modification*, (Vol. 6), 4 (1982), pp. 519–49

Meichenbaum, D. H. 'Examination of model characteristics in reducing avoidance behaviour', *Journal of Personality and Social Psychology*, 17 (1971), pp. 288–307

Mendel, J. G. C. and Klein, D. F. 'Anxiety attacks with subsequent agoraphobia', *Comprehensive Psychiatry*, 10 (1969), pp. 190–5

Mettzoff, J. and Kornreich, M. *Research in Psychotherapy*, New York, Atheuton, 1970

Miller, G. A., Galanter, E. and Pribram, K. *Plans and the Structure of Behaviour*, New York, Holt, Reinhart and Winston, 1960

Millman, H. L., Schaefer, C. E. and Cohen, J. J. (eds) *Therapies for School Behaviour Problems*, San Francisco, Jossey-Bass, 1980

Minuchin, S. and Fishman, H. C. *Family Therapy Techniques*, Cambridge, Mass., Harvard University Press, 1981

Mowrer, O. H. 'Peer groups and medication: the best "therapy" for professionals and laymen alike', *Psychotherapy: Theory Research and Practice*, 8 (1971), (1) pp. 44–5

Murray, H. A. *Explorations in Personality*, Oxford, Oxford

University Press, 1938

Naursa, M. M. 'Existential anxiety treated by systematic desensitization: A case study', *Journal of Behaviour Therapy & Experimental Psychiatry*, 2 (1971), pp. 291–5

Nemiah, J. C. 'Depersonalization neurosis', in Freedman, A. M., Kaplan, H. I. and Sadock, B. J. (eds) *Comprehensive Textbook of Psychiatry*, (vol. 1), Baltimore, Williams and Wilkins, 1975

Oakley, A. *Sex, Gender and Society*, London, Temple Smith, 1972

Ohman, A., Erikson, G. and Loftberg, I. 'Phobias and preparedness: phobic vs. neutral pictures as conditioning stimuli for human autonomic responses', *Journal of Abnormal Psychology*, 84 (1975), pp. 41–5

Ohman, A., Frederikson, M. and Hugdahl, K. 'Towards an experimental model of simple phobic reactions', *Behaviour Analysis and Modification*, 2 (1978), pp. 97–114

Ohman, A. 'Fear relevance, autonomic conditioning and phobias: a laboratory model', in Sjoden, P. O., Bates, S. and Dockens, W. S. (eds) *Trends in Behaviour Therapy*, New York, Academic Press, 1979

Paskind, H. A. 'A study of phobias', *Journal of Neurological Psychopathology*, 12 (1931), 40–6

Paul, G. L. 'Outcome of systematic desensitization II: Controlled investigation of individual treatment, technique variations and current status', in Franks, C. M. (ed.) *Behaviour Therapy Appraisal and Status*, New York, McGraw Hill, 1969

Portnoy, I. 'The anxiety states', in Arieti, S. (ed.) *American Handbook of Psychiatry*, (Vol. 1), New York, Basic Books, 1959

Prince, M. 'Clinical study of a case of phobia: A symposium', *Journal of Abnormal and Social Psychology*, 7 (1912), pp. 259–303

Proctor, H. 'Family construct psychology: an approach to understanding and treating families', in Waldron-Skinner, S. (ed.) *Developments in Family Therapy: Theories and Application since 1948*, London, Routledge and Kegan Paul, 1981

Quarentelli, E. L. 'A note on the protective function of the family in disasters', *Journal of Marriage and Family Life*, 22 (1960), pp. 263–4

Rachman, S. J. *Phobias: Their Nature and Control*, Springfield Illinois, Charles C. Thomas, 1968

Rachman, S. J. *The Meanings of Fear*, London, Penguin Books, 1974

Rachman, S. J. 'Biologically significant fears', *Behaviour Analysis and Modification*, 2 (1978), pp. 234–9

Ramsey, R. W. 'Research in anxiety and phobic reactions', in Spielberger, C. D. and Sarason, I. G. (eds), *Stress and Anxiety*, (Vol. 1), New York, John Wiley and Sons, 1975

Richter, D. 'The action of adrenaline in anxiety; *Proceedings of the*

Royal Society of Medicine, 33 (1940), pp. 615–18

Roth, H., Garside, R. S. and Gurney, C. 'Clinical-statistical enquiries into the classification of anxiety states and depressive disorders', *May and Baker conference proceedings*, Leeds, pp. 175–87, 1965

Sarbin, T. R., Taft, R. and Bailey, D. E. *Clinical Inference and Cognitive Theory*, New York, Holt, Reinhart and Winston, 1960

Schapira, K., Kerr, T. A. and Roth, M. 'Phobias and affective illness', *British Journal of Psychiatry*, 117 (1970), pp. 25–32

Seligman, M. E. P. 'Phobias and preparedness', *Behaviour Therapy*, 2 (1971), pp. 307–21

Seligman, M. E. P. and Hager, J. L. (eds) *Biological Boundaries of Learning*, New York, Appleton-Century-Crofts, 1972

Sheikh, A. A. (ed.) *Imagery*, New York, John Wiley and Sons, 1983

Shafar, S. 'Aspects of phobic illness – A study of 900 personal cases', *British Journal of Medical Psychology*, 49 (1976), pp. 211–36

Sherman, A. R. 'Real-life exposure as a primary therapeutic factor in the desensitization treatment of fear', *Journal of Abnormal Psychology*, 79 (1972), pp. 19–28

Silver, J. M. 'Competitive sports environments: Performance enhancement through cognitive intervention', *Behaviour Modification*, 1982

Sim, M. and Houghton, H. 'Phobic anxiety and its treatment', *Journal of Nervous and Mental Diseases*, 143 (1966), pp. 484–91

Slater, E. A. and Shields, J. 'Genetical aspects of anxiety', in M. Lader (ed.), 'Studies of anxiety', *British Journal of Psychiatry*, Special Publication No. 3, 1969

Slater, E. and Woodside, M. *Patterns of Marriage*, London, Tavistock, 1951

Speltz, M. L. and Bernstein, D. A. 'Sex differences in fearfulness', *Journal of Behaviour Therapy and Experimental Psychiatry*, 7 (1976), pp. 117–22

Torgerston, W. S. 'The nature and origin of common phobic fears', *British Journal of Psychiatry*, 134 (1979), pp. 343–51

Tryer, P. *The Role of Bodily Feelings in Anxiety*, Oxford, Oxford University Press, 1976

Tucker, W. I. 'Diagnosis and treatment of the phobic reaction', *American Journal of Psychiatry*, 112 (1956), pp. 825–830

Watson, J. B. and Rayner, R. 'Conditioned emotional reaction, *Journal of Experimental Psychology*, 3 (1920), pp. 1–14

Weir, S. 'The perception of motion: actions, motives and feelings', in *Progress in Perception*, University of Edinburgh Department of Artificial Intelligence Report No. 1, 1975

Wilkins, W. 'Desensitization: Social and cognitive factors, underlying the effectiveness of Wolpe's procedure', *Psychological Bulletin*, 76

(1971), pp. 311–17

Winokur, G. and Holeman, E. 'Chronic anxiety neurosis: clinical and sexual aspects', *Acta Psychiatrica Scandinavia*, 39 (1963), pp. 384–412

Wolpe, J. 'Learning Therapies', in J. G. Howels (ed.), *Modern Perspectives in World Psychiatry*, Edinburgh, Oliver and Boyd, 1968

Wolpe, J. *The Practice of Behaviour Therapy*, 2nd Ed., New York, Pergamon Press, 1973

Yates, A. J. *Behaviour Therapy*, New York, Wiley, 1970

Zuckerman, M. M. and Wheeler, L. 'To dispel fantasies about fantasy-based measure of fear of success', *Psychological Bulletin*, 82 (1975), pp. 932–46

Zung, W. W. K. 'Assessment of anxiety disorder: Qualitative and quantitative approaches', in Fann, W. E., Karacan, I., Porkorny, A. D. and Williams R. L. (eds) *Phenomenology and Treatment of Anxiety*, New York, SP Medical and Scientific Books, 1979

Index

ABC method, 64–5
achievement, need for, 55, 146–7
active imagination (relaxation
    method), 120–1
adrenaline, 31
aggression
    anxiety avoidance and, 50
    bullies and, 201, 202, 205
    red used in artwork as a sign of,
    72
agoraphobia, 11, 14
AIDS, 23, 207, 219
Allen, Woody, 211
animals, fear of, 22 *see also* cat
    phobia; dog phobia; rat phobia
ANS *see* autonomic nervous system
antecedent, noting, 64–5
anxiety
    discovering parental problems of,
        99–106
    discovering whether child suffers
        with, 61–73
    exploring causes of, 74–92
    general discussion of how to help
        children with, 109–14
    helping with specific problems,
        139–215 *see also* name of
        specific problem
    hidden fears, 42–58
    living without, 219–23
    nature of, 3–16
    pinpointing specific anxieties,
        93–8
    question about, 17–25
    reasons for occurrence of, 26–41
    relaxation response to, 115–36
arithmetic, fear of *see* maths anxiety
arms (in children's drawings), 70–1
arousal and performance
    relationship, 36, 37, 145
art, children's, 66–73, 74–7
assessing anxiety
    using artwork, 66–73, 74–7
    using checklist of statements,
        17–20, 102–6
    using diary, 64–6
    using picture assessment, 77–92
autonomic nervous system (ANS)
    child's physical and mental state
        in relation to, 31–4
    functions of, 29–30
    genetic structure and, 99, 100
    performance in relation to
        arousal of, 37
    problems posed by, 30, 35
    relaxation and, 117, 126, 128
    slow-down branch of, 30–1, 32,
        117, 126
    step-up branch of, 30–1, 32, 117,
        128
avoidance (defence mechanism)
    discussion of, 48–50
    maths, 9, 11, 158–9
    parental use of, 101, 206
    phobias and, 9, 11, 190–1
    positive aspect of, 54
    specific anxieties and, 55, 56, 57,
        58, 63, 144

banishing anxiety, practical
    procedures for, 109–36
    see also name of specific anxiety
barriers to discussion, 101–2
behaviour, noting, 65
black, use of (in children's art),
    71–2, 73
BOSS (burn-out stress syndrome),
    39
brain in relation to emotional
    responses, 35
breast size, anxiety over, 211, 212,
    213
bullying
    as major cause of anxiety, 57
    by teacher, 39–40
    case of Mike discussed, 39–40, 47
    child's fear of discussing, 46
    defence mechanisms used, 57
    discussion of problem, 201–5
    physical and mental state when
        threatened by, 31–2
burn-out stress syndrome (BOSS),
    39

calculators, 169
car travel, fear of, 65
cat phobia, 195–6
Cauthery, Philip, 213
changing-room behaviour, 16, 212,
    213
childbirth, fear of, 23
claustrophobia, 192
clothes, school, 140
clownish behaviour, 50
Cole, Martin, 213
Collins, 177
colour (in children's art), 71–3
compensations, building in, 221
compulsive behaviour, 53
consequence of behaviour, noting,
    65–6
crushes, female, 214

danger, physical response to, 26–9
    see also autonomic nervous
        system
defence mechanisms
    classroom dropouts and, 144–5
    different types of, 47–54
    maths and, 158–9
    parental use of, 100–1, 206–7
    positive value of, 54–5

used in relation to specific
    anxieties, 55, 56, 57, 58
    see also name of particular
        defence mechanism
denial of reality (defence
    mechanism), 53–4, 55, 56, 57,
    58, 101, 144, 207
diary, keeping a, 64–6
discovering anxiety
    in children, 61–73
    in parents, 99–106
    see also assessing anxiety
disguising anxiety *see* defence
    mechanisms
dismissiveness, 94–5
displacement (defence mechanism),
    51, 54, 55, 57
distortions (in children's drawings),
    68–9
distress, 36
divorce, fear of, 23
dog phobia, 11, 188, 192, 197
dominant aggressives, 201
dominant leaders, 201
dominated frightened, 201–2
Dougherty, Knowles, 163
drawing *see* art, children's

ear-shotting, 222
Effect, Law of, 189, 190
ejaculation, 209–10
emotional avoidance, 49 *see also*
    avoidance
emotional constipation, 49
emotional responses, 35
eustress, 36
exams
    case of Max discussed in relation
        to anxiety about, 8, 30, 40, 41,
        74, 101
    cause of stress, 38
    rationalisation and, 52
    rituals and, 52–3
    success in *see* exam success,
        helping achieve
exam success, helping achieve,
    171–86
    countdown to exam day, 184–6
    managing nerves, 182–4
    managing time, 174–7
    planning for, 171–4
    studying, 177–82
    see also exams

exercise, 154
exploring child's anxieties, 74–92
extroverts, 21, 99–100
Eysenck, Dr Hans, 21

failure
  as means of reducing fear, 144–5
  fear of, 6, 23, 55, 143–4, 146–52
family feelings, fears about, 56
family influence, 112
fantasy training, 152, 194, 196–7,
    198, 199, 204–5 *see also* Mind
    Movies
fear, general discussion of
  hidden, 42–58
  nature of, 9–10
  questions about, 21–4
  see also anxiety; names of specific
    fears and anxieties
Fearless Tiger, 119, 132–3, 196,
    199, 205, 219
fight or flee responses, 26–8
Floppy Bear, 119, 131–2, 219
flying, phobia about, 198
foreign languages, learning, 178
formulae, learning, 178
Fox, Dr Cynthia, 70
Freud, 24, 51, 52, 96, 188, 211
friendship, anxieties about, 3, 63,
    89–90, 113 *see also* social
    anxiety

genetic factors, 20–1, 41, 99–100
'getting it over with' strategy, 9 *see
    also* impulsive behaviour
ghosts, fear of, 22, 23
GIGO (Garbage In, Garbage Out)
    remarks, 150
Gillies, Pam, 23
goals set in treatment of phobias,
    192–3, 194–5, 196, 197, 199
Gray, Thomas, 145
Greek mathematicians, 169–70
green, use of (in children's art), 73
guessing (in maths), 168–9

Handler, Dr Leonard, 66
hands (in children's drawings),
    70–1
Happy Hound, 119, 133, 199
health
  affected by anxiety, 4, 6, 17, 38,
    39, 64

exams and, 184
fears about, 57
heavy pressure (in children's
    drawings), 69–70
Heim, Alice, 49
helping anxious children
  practical procedures for, 109–36
  with specific problems, 139–215
  see also name of specific
    problem
hidden fears, 42–58
  case study, 42–4
  causes of anxiety, 55–8
  methods of disguising anxiety,
    47–55
  reasons why children hide
    anxiety, 44–7
Holmes, F. B., 21
homework, helping with, 152–5
homosexual attraction, 101, 207,
    213–14
hospital, anxiety about, 67–8
human figures, drawings of, 66–73,
    75–6

ideogram, 176, 182
imaginary fears, 23
immune system, 38
impotence, 207
impulsive behaviour, 9, 49–50
independence, encouragement of,
    213
influence, zones of, 111–13
intellectual ability, teachers'
    judgement of, 145–6
intellectual achievement, anxiety
    and, 23–4, 34–5, 62–3 *see also*
    school anxiety
intellectual avoidance, 48 *see also*
    avoidance
interplay between people, 109–13
interviews, fear of, 197
introverts, 21, 99
island of peace, 126–8

Jerslid, Arthur T., 21

Kinsey, 213
knowledge networks, 177–82
Kripke, Saul, 159

latency stage (in learning maths), 167
Law of Effect, 189, 190

Lazarus, Mitchell, 167
Leibnitz, 170
listening, 68, 89, 93–8
Little Albert, 187
living without anxiety, 219–23

masturbation, 40, 207, 213
maths anxiety
  avoidance and, 9, 11, 48, 158–9
  case of Alison discussed, 62
  helping to overcome, 159–70
  widespread occurrence of, 155,
    156–8
  meeting grown-ups' expectations,
    55, 90
menstruation, 209, 210
mental symptoms of anxiety *see*
  symptoms, anxiety
Mind Movies
  dealing with exams, 171, 182–3,
    184, 186
  dealing with phobias, 191, 194,
    196–7, 199
  dealing with school anxiety, 152
  dealing with social anxiety, 205
  technique for creating, 125–30
misinformation, correcting, 219
mock situations, 197–8
modelling, 100
monsters, fear of, 22, 23
Montagner, Professor Hubert, 201
mother, phobia about, 14
mouths (in children's drawings),
  70–1
muscle-focusing (relaxation
  method), 122–5

negative numbers, 167, 170
new situations, coping with, 91 *see
  also* unknown, anxiety about
nuclear war, fears about, 23, 57–8,
  113
nudity, public, 16, 210–13

observation (to identify anxiety),
  64–6
omissions (in children's drawings),
  67–8
orgasm, female, 207
overpainting, 73
overstress *see* stress

painting *see* art, children's

panic attack, 33, 34
parapraxes, 96
parents
  assessment of own anxieties,
    99–106
  communication of anxieties, 20–1
  dealing with own phobia, 198
  importance of role, 24–5, 112,
    195–6
  improving mathematical
    knowledge, 160–1
  problems in discussing sexual
    anxiety, 101, 206–7
  rejection by, 46–7
  see also meeting grown-ups'
    expectations
patience, need for, 222
Peak Performance Stress Level
  (PPSL), 37, 145
penis size, anxiety over, 207,
  211–12, 213
performance and arousal
  relationship, 36, 37, 145
persistence, need for, 222
personal training plan, creating, 16
phobias
  case of spider phobia *see* spider
    phobia, discussion of case of
  children's strategies for dealing
    with, 9
  development of, 48, 100, 113,
    187–91
  helping phobic child, 187–200
  problems described, 3, 10–14
  programme for banishing,
    191–200
  symptom substitution and, 24
  types of, 9, 11–13
physical imperfections, adolescent
  concern about, 211
physical injury, fear of, 22, 23
physical response to danger, 26–9
  see also autonomic nervous
    system
physical symptoms of anxiety
  see health: affected by anxiety,
    physical response to danger
    symptoms, anxiety
picture assessment, 77–92
PIN approach, 149
pinpointing specific anxieties, 93–8
positive attitude, need for, 222
positive listening *see* listening

poverty, fear of, 23
PPSL (Peak Performance Stress Level), 37, 145
praise, 149, 195, 222
privacy, need for, 211, 212
procedure, errors of mathematical, 161–3
professional help, 24
projection (defence mechanism), 50–1, 55, 56, 57, 144, 158, 206
projective test (picture assessment), 77–92
prudence, need for, 222
puberty
  average age for different stages of, 209
  preparation for, 209
  stress and, 38
public nudity, anxiety over, 16, 210–13
public speaking, anxiety over, 197–8
punishments, 149–50
puppet dance (relaxation method), 121–2
purple, use of (in children's art), 71–2, 73

questions about anxiety answered, 17–25
Quillan, 177

rating anxiety, 193–4
rationalisation (defence mechanism), 52, 54, 55, 56, 58, 63, 101, 144, 158, 206
rat phobia, 187
red, use of (in children's art), 72, 73
regression, 220
rejection, 46–7
relaxation in relation to specific anxiety problems
  exams, 171, 182, 184, 186
  phobias, 191, 194, 198–9
  social anxiety, 204
  see also relaxation response
relaxation response, 115–36
  difficulties encountered, 128, 130
  images to help younger children, 131–3
  Mind Movies, 125–8
  rapid relaxation, 130
  teaching children physical relaxation, 117–25

tension, 115–17
  see also relaxation in relation to specific anxiety problems
repression (defence mechanism), 51, 54–5, 56, 57, 58
revision, exam, 171–4, 175, 179–81, 184
rewards, 149–50, 189–90, 199
Reyger, Dr Joseph, 66
rituals, 52–3
rules, anxiety about following, 140

same-sex attraction, 101, 207, 213–14
school anxiety
  case studies, 39–40, 62–3, 94, 153, 221
  children branded as stupid, 145–6
  compensations and, 221
  discussion about helping child with, 139–55
  failure as means of reducing fears, 144–5
  fantasy training, 152
  fear of failure, 146–52
  homework, 152–5
  mentioned, 3, 22
  need for achievement, 146–7
  phobia, 11, 221
  picture assessment, 89
  projection as defence mechanism, 50–1
  school as zone of influence, 112
  starting school, 38, 139–41
  stressful periods, 38
  talking to teachers, 141–3
self-defeating talk, avoiding, 159–60
self-esteem, boosting, 222
self-image, 5, 111–12, 150, 221
self-mockery, 96
Selye, Dr Hans, 36
separation, anxiety over, 22, 141
Sewell, Bridget, 156, 157
sex education, 206, 208–10
sexual abuse, 45–6
sexual anxiety
  causes of, 56–7
  children's fear of admitting, 45–6
  common among teenagers, 23
  defence mechanisms and, 57
  helping with, 206–15
  parental problems in discussing, 101, 206–7
  repression and, 51

sexual inadequacy, worry about, 211–12
Sidis, William James, 159
slips of the tongue, 96
slow-down mechanism of ANS, 30–1, 32, 117, 126
social anxiety, 3, 201–5 *see also* bullying
society, influence of, 113
Solzhenitsyn, Alexander, 160–1
spider phobia, discussion of case of problems, 7, 30, 40–1, 45, 47, 61, 74
treatment, 7, 24, 192, 194–5, 196
sport, 3, 15, 204
state anxiety, definition of, 99
step-up mechanism of ANS, 30–1, 32, 117, 128
strangers, fear of, 22, 23
stress, 36–9, 40, 148
study techniques, 177–82
success, attitudes to, 55
   see also achievement, need for; failure, fear of
symptoms, anxiety
   anxiety assessment and, 91
   list of, 10
   need to understand reasons for, 14–15
   see also autonomic nervous system; fight or flee response
symptom substitution, 24

targets set in treatment of phobias, 192–3, 194–5, 196, 197, 199
teachers
   bulling by, 39–40
   talking to, 141–3
teenage anxieties, 22–3, 113 *see also* sexual anxiety

Teevan, Dr Richard, 148
television, 153–4
tension, 115–17, 183
time allocation
   for exam questions, 174–7
   for revision, 172–4, 175
Tobias, Sheila, 157, 159, 167
'trait' anxiety, 21, 99–100
traumatic experience, 24
truancy, 48, 56

understress, 36, 37
undoing (defence mechanism), 52–3, 55, 144
unemployment, fear of, 23, 113
unfamiliar situations, coping with 91 *see also* unknown, anxiety about
unknown, anxiety about, 139–40 *see also* unfamiliar situations, coping with

vagina, masculine, 207–8
VD, 207
violence, fears about, 57–8, 113

Warren, Joseph, 169
Watson, John Broadus, 187
Watson, Dr Murray, 28–9
wet dreams, 45
words, errors over mathematical, 166–7

Yamamoto, Dr Kaoru, 149
yellow, use of (in children's art), 73

zero, problems with mathematical concept of, 163–6, 169–70